Contents

/

All King's Fund publications can be ordered from:
BEBC, PO Box 1496, Poole, Dorset BH12 3YD,
or can be purchased in person from the King's
Fund Bookshop, 11–13 Cavendish Square,
London W1M 0AN

Acknowledgements

The author and the King's Fund wish to thank all those who have contributed to this publication, either by telling their stories or by commenting on the text.

The author would also like to thank Roma Iskander and Barbara Vaughan of the King's Fund Nursing Developments Programme for their interest and support.

The author

Nancy Kohner is a writer, trainer and researcher working on a range of health and social issues. She has a particular interest in the experiences and needs of patient/client groups and in practice and policy development within the health service.

Nancy writes for both professional and lay audiences. Her books for the general public include *Having a Baby* (BBC Books, 1988), *Caring at Home* (National Extension College, 1992), and *What Shall We Tell the Children?* (BBC Books, 1993), all distributed in conjunction with successful BBC television series; and *When a Baby Dies* (Harper Collins, 2nd edition, 1995) co-written with Alix Henley. Her work for health care professionals includes a number of books which have contributed to service development and change: for example, *Pregnancy Loss and the Death of a Baby. Guidelines for Professionals* (SANDS, revised edition, 1995); *Pregnancy Loss and the Death of a Baby. A Training Pack for Professionals* (National Extension College, 1995) co-written with Ali Leftwich; and for the King's Fund Nursing Developments Programme, *Clinical Supervision in Practice* (King's Fund, 1994).

Nancy also works with organisations and health care professionals as a consultant and trainer. She has particular expertise in the area of loss and grief and provides professional training in this and related subject areas.

A note on terms

For the purposes of this publication, the terms 'ethics' and 'morality' are used interchangeably. Where one is chosen in preference to the other, it is because of style and usage rather than meaning.

The terms 'patient', 'client' and 'user' all occur. Where nurses used these words in their story-telling, the words they chose have been reproduced. Elsewhere in the text, 'user' generally refers to the consumer of the service, whereas 'patient' and 'client' are generally used to describe the individual person receiving care.

'Nurse' is intended, where appropriate, to include midwives and health visitors in both hospital and community settings.

Introduction

This publication has two main purposes:

- to help nurses and other health care workers develop an awareness and understanding of ethics in nursing practice in general, and in their own practice in particular;
- to prompt and facilitate reflection and discussion on ethical issues in day-to-day practice.

Based on practitioners' stories, it also has a practical purpose. It aims to reveal, by an exploration of nurses' experiences, the fundamentally moral nature of health care and to demonstrate the importance of ethical thinking in everyday practice. The text makes little direct reference to ethical theories. It takes its themes from nurses' own experiences, and in discussing those themes, attempts to recognise and reflect the intimate relationship between ethics and practice. Theoretical discussion is readily available elsewhere, and some texts are suggested on pages 90–2.

The background to this publication lies in a small project initiated by the King's Fund Nursing Developments Programme, designed to document and explore nurses' experiences of ethical difficulty in their day-to-day practice. Informal interviews were carried out in a number of NDUs around the country, sometimes with individual nurses, sometimes with small groups. The purpose of these interviews was to gather stories about ethical dilemmas and difficulties, and in particular to listen to these stories as they were related by the nurses involved. The intention was to focus not only on the nature of, and reasons for, ethical difficulty but also on nurses' experiences, asking them to reflect on what they thought and felt and on what their experiences meant for them professionally and personally.

The nurses who contributed these stories were all interested in developing their ideas about ethical practice. All, for example, were concerned about the difficulties they faced in trying to give high quality, individual care and to protect and respect the rights of their patients or clients. None, however, was specifically engaged in work on ethical issues; none possessed particular expertise in this area, and most agreed that their training not only lacked formal input on ethics but also neglected in a more general sense the ethical dimension of nursing practice. They recognised ethics to be pervasive in their work and considered ethical thinking to be important in developing their practice. They commented that they lacked, yet would value, opportunities to consider and debate ethical concerns.

The stories that they told, along with supplementary material gathered from other sources, are therefore offered in this publication as material for discussion and reflection. Each story is followed by suggested discussion points, and each group of stories is followed by a brief commentary (Chapter 1). Chapter 2 (page 55) identifies key factors in the development of ethical practice, and Chapter 3 (page 57) suggests ways in which ethical thinking can be practised and developed.

Stories of ethical difficulty in nursing practice

'Hospitals are ethical minefields in terms of the daylight robbery of people's rights and dignity that goes on from the instant they walk in at the door.'

'It's true that hospitals are ethical minefields. But there is no barbed wire and no signposts.'

(Two nurses involved in group discussion about ethics in nursing practice)

'Even going into people's homes you hold the power. It's easy to forget that.'

(A health visitor)

The nurses who told the stories in this chapter were simply asked to recall ethical difficulties they had experienced in their day-to-day work. They were offered no prior definitions of either ethics or ethical practice. In fact, nurses asked to produce a story about a specific ethical issue – say, confidentiality or truth-telling – could rarely do so. The stories are simply those that sprang to mind at the time of the interview as difficult experiences, and they therefore reflect the nurses' own ideas about ethics in health care and their feelings about what is ethically difficult in their practice.

The result is a diverse collection of accounts, yet in all the stories there is a common theme, or a common and over-arching problem. It is the nurses' commitment to care for clients *as people* that leads them inevitably and directly into ethical conflict or difficulty.

3

Caring for clients as people is not a new concept in health care policy. The Government's manifesto for community care, *Caring for People,*[1] specifies that a key component of community care should be services that respond flexibly and sensitively to the needs of individuals and their carers. *The Patient's Charter,*[2] launched in 1991 under the banner of 'putting patients first', is an explicit attempt to give health service users some rights, respect and power. In 1993, *A Vision for the Future,*[3] looking at the future of nursing, midwifery and health visiting, makes the development of individualised patient care its first target and describes new initiatives in nursing as resulting in 'an understanding of each individual, and a desire to participate with them in their health care in a way that preserves their dignity.' *Changing Childbirth,*[4] describing a new policy for the maternity services, states as its first principle that the individual woman 'must be the focus of maternity care. She should be able to feel that she is in control of what is happening to her and able to make decisions about her care . . .'

At the same time, developments in nursing practice, such as primary nursing, the named-nurse initiative, continuity of care and advocacy, have also contributed to the widespread acceptance of the desirability of individualised care, and have mapped the way in which such care can, or should, be administered. These developments have taken place in the wider context of the growth of consumerism in health care and, more widely still, an increasing emphasis on individual freedoms in society at large.

Nevertheless, in policy and practice development alike, relatively little attention has been paid to the moral principles and values which underpin the concept – and should inform the practice – of individualised nursing care. Although links are made between ethical concepts (such as autonomy) and the art of nursing practice, thorough and reflective exploration of the meaning of these concepts in the everyday work of the ordinary practitioner is still perhaps lacking outside textbooks on health care ethics. This publication offers a starting point.

The stories told in this chapter do not constitute a comprehensive survey of the ethics of individualised care. They are a random collection of accounts which illustrate a variety of ethical difficulties, some dramatic, others mundane and seemingly trivial, but all significant. They can be roughly grouped in four broad categories, each of which represents an important aspect of caring for clients as people:

I. Accepting and respecting the individuality and autonomy of the patient or client

II. The nurse-patient/client relationship

III. The nurse-family relationship

IV. The role and responsibilities of the nurse

There are overlaps between these categories and most stories illustrate difficulties of more than one kind. It is almost inevitable, for example, that difficulties within the nurse-client relationship will also raise questions about the role and responsibilities of the nurse; and that difficulties to do with respect for a client's autonomy should raise questions about the nurse-client relationship. Nevertheless, these groupings provide a focus for discussion and allow links and comparisons to be made between different experiences of ethical difficulty.

The stories are reproduced as they were told, with some editing for the sake of clarity and style. This means that the stories, and the difficulties they describe, remain personal and real, and it is likely that many nurses will find accounts of experiences very similar to their own. The intention is to demonstrate and emphasise that ethics is an integral part of practice, and to relate the consideration and discussion of ethical issues not only to the realities of day-to-day care but also to nurses' experiences of care-giving.

The stories encourage identification: most nurses, midwives and health visitors have similar stories to tell. Even so, some stories are likely to provoke a critical response in many readers. It is sometimes easier to read objectively and to distance the experience than to identify with it, and it is certainly easy to respond to a story by saying 'She shouldn't have done that' or 'He should have done this'. It may be important to set these reactions aside and to recognise the stories as commonly shared experiences.

It is also important to bear in mind that the stories represent only the nurses' perspective. Other health care professionals would almost certainly have different viewpoints. More importantly, this publication does not offer comparable stories from patients and clients and therefore only half the story is told. This is a significant omission, and in Chapter 3 (page 57), the importance of hearing users' stories is discussed.

Each group of stories is followed by a brief commentary, drawing out some common themes and questions. Although discussion of the stories could be focused around specific ethical theories, or could be used to develop the use of ethical frameworks (as suggested, for example, by Seedhouse[5]), the aim here is to offer some starting points for reflection on the ethical questions that the stories raise. The stories are not intended as problem-solving exercises but as devices to allow the development of ethical awareness and thinking.

For further suggestions about facilitating discussion around these stories, see Chapter 3 (page 57).

I Accepting and respecting the individuality and autonomy of the patient or client

Story 1 Against her wishes

'There's one patient we looked after recently who'd been in the special care unit for some time. It got to the stage where she was able to express herself and she was able to indicate whether she did or didn't want care. And she made it quite clear that she didn't want nursing care. She didn't want to be washed or turned or anything like that. And there was a dilemma, because we could either adhere to the patient's wishes or we could give her the physical care she needed. I could see she just wanted to be left in peace really, but I thought as well she seemed quite hopeless and depressed and I wondered whether the fact she didn't want anything done for her was to do with those feelings.

'I tried to give her as much choice as possible. After all, not being washed wasn't going to harm her, so if she didn't want to be washed, she wasn't washed. But obviously there was quite a lot we went on doing for her which was against her wishes. We just tried at the same time to give her a lot of reassurance and support so that she could see some hope in her situation. It was difficult and I don't know that we always got the balance right.'

Discussion points

- What reasons (if any) might there be for not agreeing to a patient's requests or wishes?

- How do you think you might feel as a patient if you asked for something and were denied it?

- Do patients have the right to dictate the care they are given? If not, why not?

- Do patients have the right to refuse care and/or treatment?

- How would you feel if a patient refused care that you felt was in their best interests?

Story 2 'Get me home'

'I was involved in the care of a lady who came in with very severe heart failure. She made a tremendous recovery against all the odds and she was determined to go home, but her continuing recovery was going to depend on compliance with two very important things. One was taking the tablets that she'd been prescribed, and the other was not drinking more than about two and a half pints of fluid a day.

'Now this lady could do very little and didn't have much left to enjoy in life, but one thing she did enjoy was making lots of pots of tea. And she probably used to drink about eight to ten, maybe even more, cups of tea a day. Added to that, she didn't like taking her tablets. All she saw was a lot of tablets she had to take and she couldn't relate taking the tablets to actually feeling better. So her perception was, "I don't really like taking the tablets and I do like my cups of tea."

'Just to make the situation even more difficult, this lady was profoundly deaf, so she couldn't hear the doorbell, and she'd been broken into in the past, so she was terrified of opening the front door. The community staff knew this lady and they knew they wouldn't be able to get into the house to visit her.

'So this was the background against which we had to look at her discharge. For us it was very problematic, but all this lady knew was "Get me home".'

Discussion points

- Does the patient have a right to be discharged, even if this involves risk?

- What is the extent of a nurse's responsibility to protect a patient from harm?

- What could you do in this situation in order to meet the woman's need to go home and yet minimise risk?

Story 3 'Tell me what to do'

'I've known this family for about seven years now. I met Anne when she had her first baby and I was her health visitor. That first baby had a different father, but she met Sean when the baby was a few months old and they got together about that time. He was a lovely man but he never had a job in the time I knew him and there was a lot of stress and difficulty, financial and otherwise. Anne had three more babies in the space of the next five years and about two months ago she arrived at the clinic and told me she was pregnant again and that Sean had left her.

'She looked dreadful. She was worn out for a start and really not well. The relationship with Sean had been going downhill for a long time. I knew that because obviously I'd seen her a lot and we'd got to know each other quite well. I felt I'd got a good relationship with her but I also felt very frustrated because I couldn't do much to help.

'She said she wanted the baby, but a week later I saw her at home and she said she'd thought about it and she just couldn't see her way to having it and caring for it, so she was going to arrange a termination. I supported her in that, and anyway, I felt it was the right decision. She wasn't coping at all.

'Then about two weeks after that I saw her again and she hadn't arranged the termination. She was very tearful and unhappy and she said she just couldn't make her mind up what to do. I tried to help her think it through again but it was very difficult. I could see how torn she was. I found it hard to be unbiased because the truth was I felt she shouldn't have the baby. Anyway, in the end she turned to me and said, "I can't decide. Tell me what to do." She said all she wanted was to have the decision made and she couldn't make it herself. She just needed somebody to make it for her.'

Discussion points

● Should the health visitor give advice or should she hold back, saying it has to be Anne's decision? Give your reasons.

● The health visitor knows Anne's personal situation and has an established and good relationship with her. Are there factors that might justify her expressing an opinion about what Anne should do? Would your thinking about the situation change if the health visitor did not know Anne well?

● What might be the short- and long-term consequences of the health visitor giving, or not giving, advice?

● In what circumstances, if any, should a health professional make a decision on a client's behalf?

● Do you think that Sean has any rights in this situation?

Story 4 'She never asked . . .'

'A girl came to us who was just 19. She had quite a vicious cancer that was growing extremely quickly. She'd had a very short time between experiencing her first problem and coming to the specialised unit. She was here for about a week for investigations.

'We told her parents that we couldn't cure the cancer, that we knew we couldn't cure it, but we could give some treatment that hopefully would help. But they said no, because some very close friends of theirs had a son who'd been treated here, and he'd gone through more than 12 months of very intense chemotherapy and then he'd died. He'd had chemotherapy, he'd had surgery, but it just didn't control his disease at all and he died. So this girl's parents equated treatment with a lot of needless suffering.

'It was very difficult because we are quite good at palliative care here. And it was distressing to have somebody so young and so desperately ill and for her parents to be not only against giving any treatment (which I can understand) but also against giving her any information. So she didn't know that she was going to die. And it's so strange, because normally we don't go with what relatives want. We just say very clearly that we'll always be honest with somebody and that we feel they need information.

'I used to spend a little bit of time with the girl and I can remember thinking, "Well, she never asked me any questions . . ." I think I was kidding myself that she'd had the chance to ask questions but hadn't asked any. When the truth was, I didn't particularly want to get into a conversation with her. Normally, we would give information to any patient, no matter what age, but with this girl, we were very reluctant. And some of it was because her parents were so against her being told, being hurt, being treated. They were an articulate couple, able to speak their minds very clearly and tell you exactly how they felt. They weren't aggressive, just very down-to-earth, very balanced.'

Discussion points

- Do you consider the nurse's agreement not to give the girl information about her illness is justifiable? On what grounds?

- Do patients have a right to know that they are dying?

- Suppose the nurse had decided to tell the girl that she was dying. What might the consequences have been? Consider both the girl's possible feelings and her parents'.

- This nurse's response might have been different if she had found the girl's parents less sympathetic. How much is practice influenced by positive or negative feelings about patients/clients and their families? Is it right that it should be influenced in this way?

Story 5 An open door

'Like many wards with patients with dementia, the door here is kept locked. The cleaner, who is often near the door, is repeatedly asked by patients to let them out. And she will lie to them and say, "I can't open the door." She has no problem with that.

'But people's feelings about wanting to get through that door, and feeling trapped when they can't, are valid feelings and we have to look at what we can do about it.

'So if a patient rattles at the door, we open the door and walk out with him. Maybe he'll go a short distance up the corridor and then get tired and we'll come back together and sit down and have a cup of tea. Maybe we'll go further. You can have quite a pleasant walk round the grounds for 20 or 25 minutes. Occasionally, if people feel the need for cigarettes, they might be escorted out of the ward and up the road to the petrol station. It gets them out of the unit and it's also a way of assessing their abilities.

'A patient might want to go home. So a nurse might have to go out with that patient and catch a bus and go to the patient's home. But isn't that a more constructive use of that nurse's time than working with the patient on the ward dissuading him or her from trying to leave? The same amount of time can be used on the ward as off it, and the bus ride builds the relationship whereas fighting damages it.'

Discussion points

- What are your feelings about responding to patients in this way?

- If a patient asks to leave the ward, on what grounds can you justify not allowing him or her to do so? How do you feel about this justification?

- If a patient asks to leave the ward and is prevented from doing so, what does this mean for the nurse—patient relationship?

How does the nurse–patient relationship change if the door is opened and the patient is accompanied out?

● Are there any considerations to be taken into account besides the rights and needs of the patients?

Story 6 Permissible or indefensible?

'On an acute medical ward, the minute you have an empty bed, you have people coming in through the door, and you just don't know what's going to come, and it can dramatically affect the whole ward, it can put everything out. I remember one day a guy coming in through the door who was very psychotic but who was also profoundly physically ill. But he was not so ill that he couldn't march up and down the ward – a big, imposing guy, knocking over the crash trolley, playing with the defibrillator, threatening physical violence and really scaring the other patients. He was causing absolute mayhem.

'Well, later he was put on a section but before that I just knew that we had to get this guy to calm down. And there was absolutely no way we could wait while we got all the right people in the right place to do the section. It was a general hospital, so there was always delay while we phoned the local psychiatric hospital and so on. So he was prescribed sedation, but he simply couldn't see that he needed it. And I felt I had to give it to him in some way, so I put it in his tea.

'But it's interesting for me remembering that now, because at the moment a relative of mine is in hospital and he is being chemically restrained because he is being aggressive. He's being aggressive not because he's in any way demented or incompetent or anything like that but because he's angry. He's absolutely furious. He's been put into hospital, he can't see very well, he can't hear very well, he's elderly and debilitated. And the nurses are pulling him around and changing his whole day-to-day routine and they're not listening to him and he hit out with his stick. So the nurses asked for a drug to be prescribed and they're giving it to him. But they're not giving him any choice about it: they're putting it in his tea. And my response to this is outrage. I think it's appalling.'

Discussion points

- Do you consider that tranquillising patients without their knowledge or consent can be justified? On what grounds?

- Following an incident like this, what could nurses on the ward do to avoid or mitigate similar difficulties in the future?

- This nurse's feelings as a relative were very different to his feelings as a professional. How might his feelings as a relative influence his professional practice in the future?

Story 7 Duty or interference?

'I remember a guy coming in one night obviously drunk and he'd driven to Accident and Emergency.

'This chap had been a bit abusive but no more than you'd expect on a normal Saturday night. And he got back in his car after we'd finished with him and off he went.

'It happened that the husband of the sister on duty was a traffic bobby, and she knew where he was working that particular night. This sister went to the phone and rang her husband and gave him the registration number of the car. So she turned him in.

'I didn't agree with it at the time, and if she'd discussed it with me I think I would have told her not to do it. But afterwards I thought long and hard about it. There was the question of the man's own life, but he could also have damaged or even killed someone else. What was our responsibility in that situation?'

Discussion points

- Do you consider it was right or wrong of the nurse to pass on this information? Give your reasons.

- Consider and decide how you would act in this situation. Give your reasons.

Commentary: Accepting and respecting the autonomy of the individual patient or client

The underlying moral principle of individual or client-centred care is the acceptance of, and respect for, the autonomy of the individual. Not only the stories in this group but most of the stories in this publication raise questions to do with personal autonomy.

An autonomous person may be described as someone who is able to choose for him or herself and be self-determining. Seedhouse [5] describes autonomy as 'a person's capacity to choose freely for himself, and to be able to direct his own life'. Gillon [6] describes autonomy as 'deliberated self-rule', that is, the ability to make our own decisions on the basis of deliberation.

If respect for autonomy is accepted as a moral imperative of health care, other imperatives follow. In practice, respecting the autonomy of the individual patient or client would seem to demand:

- giving information
- communication (including listening)
- offering choice
- meeting the client's expressed wishes
- obtaining informed consent
- honesty
- confidentiality
- non–judgemental care
- dignity for the client.

(Respect for autonomy does not necessarily demand patient participation, although these two ideas are frequently linked and sometimes confused. Respect for autonomy may involve respecting a client's choice *not* to participate in his or her care, or to participate only in certain ways or to a certain extent. It may also involve respecting a decision not to be informed and/or not to exercise choice.)

However, it is in the practical application of the principle of respect for autonomy, through the kind of care the words listed above describe, that ethical difficulties are most likely to arise. Stories in this chapter illustrate some of these difficulties.

Theoretically, it could be argued that the best way to respect another's autonomy is simply to leave them alone, not to interfere or intervene. However, if someone is ill, hurt or otherwise in need of care, others will wish to help. This too is a matter of moral principle. For the health professional, it is also a professional duty – and a job. So how can a professional help – or intervene – in a way that still respects, as far as possible, the autonomy of the person in need of care?

This question is complicated by the fact that the relationship between a carer and a person cared for is fundamentally unequal. When the caregiver is a professional, the inequality is greater. Illness or need creates vulnerability and dependency; medical knowledge and caring skills confer power. It will be difficult to show respect for the person needing care and accord them the autonomy to which they are entitled unless some steps are taken to redress the imbalance in the professional-client relationship.

The way in which health care is organised exacerbates the problem. For example, the hospital as an institution increases the dependency and vulnerability of those who need its services. Patients' lives within hospital are severely constrained, not simply by the necessities of treatment but also by the institutional environment and the systems by which the hospital is run. Care that takes place outside hospital is similarly governed by systems, and those who are ignorant of these systems or, for whatever reason, cannot or do not wish to comply with them, are disadvantaged. Professionals, on the other hand, are empowered by their familiarity with health care institutions and systems, even though they may also be constrained by them.

The question of how to provide care yet at the same time respect an individual's autonomy has no clear or simple answer. It is possible, however, to devise practical approaches to the problem by means of ethical thinking. What has to be decided, in this as in most moral decisions, is not what is absolutely right or wrong, moral or immoral, but rather what is *most right* or *most moral*. While individuals will adopt

I Accepting and respecting the
individuality and autonomy
of the patient or client

different moral stances according to their own values and beliefs (and
self-awareness is therefore vital), responsible decisions cannot be made
subjectively, and careful consideration of the ethical issues is essential.

The first factor to be considered is the patient's or client's desire to
be helped and the acceptability of the help that is offered, since in
moral terms it must be considered *dis*respectful to the client to give
care that is not wanted. An important key, therefore, to the provision of
individual care is giving choice. Only by giving choice, and accepting
and implementing the choices that are made, can the caregiver know
whether the care given is acceptable, or indeed whether it should be
given it at all. Equally important, nurses must also be prepared and able
to listen and respond to voluntarily expressed needs and wishes. Good
communication, the sharing of information (on which choices can be
based), and obtaining consent are all implicated.

There is no difficulty in giving choice if a nurse's assessment of a
client's needs, and of the kind of care that should be given, coincides
with the client's own views and wishes. (Nor is there *apparently* a
problem if a client does not express, for whatever reason, any views or
wishes at all, although this situation, which may hold hidden conflict,
is worrying and uncomfortable.) However, where there is disagreement
between the client and the nurse, difficulties arise which centre on the
rights of the client to influence or decide his or her own care. The
decisive question is: is it ever justifiable to give care or treatment that a
patient expressly does not want? If so, on what grounds?

In Story 1 (page 7), a patient in intensive care states clearly that she
does not want any nursing care. The nurse attempts to meet the
patient's wishes as far as she can. The nurse feels, for example, that it will
not harm the patient not to be washed. But the nurse finds herself
unable to meet the patient's request in full. She continues to give some
care, knowing that this is against the patient's wishes. For her, this is the
'most moral' compromise she is able to reach, but she comments that,
because it is a compromise, she continues to feel uncertain about it.

Story 9 (page 25) presents the converse situation: care that is
requested is withheld. During the late stages of labour, a midwife
decides to ignore her client's request for an epidural. Unlike the nurse
in Story 1, the midwife has had the chance to develop a relationship
with her client through the months of her pregnancy and has discussed
pain relief with her antenatally. The client has said clearly, in advance

of labour, that she does not want an epidural. Does this justify the midwife's decision not to give an epidural when the woman asks for one? Do her prior discussions with her client and her professional knowledge of women in labour make her situation significantly different from the nurse working in intensive care?

There is, of course, power involved in the exercise of choice. Giving choice is to give power – and, inevitably, to surrender power too, since the professional must then accept and, if necessary, implement the choice that the client makes. Yet it may be that the client makes a choice that the professional considers unwise or wrong. More difficult still, the client may make a choice that the professional knows would be harmful and possibly even fatal. Must the choice still be accepted, or are there justifiable limits to be placed around a patient's right to make decisions about his or her treatment or care? Should the door of a dementia ward, for example, be kept locked, and patients refused the right to walk out of the door when they ask to do so? In Story 5 (page 12), nurses make a decision to open the door and accompany patients who wish to go out.

In Story 2 (page 8), an elderly woman expresses a desire to return home from hospital after a severe illness. It seems unlikely that she will be able to care for herself properly, and discharging her may put her at risk, but she is determined to go home. Does the *UKCC Code of Professional Conduct*,[7] which requires nurses to safeguard patients and clients, make the denial of choice and power legitimate – and even necessary – in a situation like this?

In the story in question, the nurse did not think so and resolved the difficulty in this way:

'We try to support the patient in what they want, even if it's inherently risky, because we believe that people have those rights. The major principle within the UKCC Code is that you will not do harm to patients or bring harm about. But to my mind even the notion of doing harm is not always clear-cut and you can't actually constrain someone who is perfectly capable of making their own decisions, even if their decisions seem entirely perverse.

'I think the important thing is to try to be guided by principles but also to look at the particular situation. Here's a lady who makes lots of cups of tea. Now, what can you actually do to try and improve that in some way? Well, you can accept that this is a lady who likes the comfort of having a nice hot

drink. Fine. But can you negotiate with her to use a smaller cup? Can you negotiate with her to use a smaller pot? Or to make tea by the cup? Can you suggest that she has as many cups of tea as she likes but maybe only takes a few mouthfuls?

'*There are other things. This lady was scared of people getting into her house so she didn't want to leave the door off the latch. But would she be happy for the district nurses to have a key? And then there are all sorts of alarms and intercoms . . .*

'*So part of it is not to accept things at face value but to negotiate. How can you make it so that the person doesn't feel as though they have lost everything, but at the same time you feel you have limited the risk?*'

This nurse reaches a similar compromise to the nurse in Story 1 (page 7). However, in some circumstances, compromise may not seem possible. Particularly challenging questions about possible limits to individual autonomy are raised when a person is very vulnerable. In Story 18 (page 46), a nurse acts to prevent a patient committing suicide, deliberately denying the woman's autonomy in (as the nurse judges) her best interests. The nurse explains her rationale:

'*I think I decided I didn't want her to die, because I thought that she was mentally ill and it was her mental illness that was making her want to die. I also knew that she really loved her children and they really loved her and I felt that I had to help to keep her alive for her children.*'

In less extreme circumstances, what kind of rationale (if any) would be sufficient to justify the denial of autonomy? In Story 17 (page 45), a woman with a mild learning disability is potentially at risk in her relationship with the taxi driver who takes her to and from a bingo session each week. Is her vulnerability sufficient reason to justify intervention of some kind in a very private part of her life? If, as Gillon[6] suggests, autonomy means the ability to make our own decisions on the basis of deliberation, does a limited capacity to deliberate limit our autonomy? Stories 6 and 7 (pages 13 and 14) tell of patients that are drunk and psychotic. Do these patients have less right to autonomy, or perhaps a right to a lesser degree of autonomy, because of their condition? And if so, who judges and decides how much autonomy they should have, and how?

All these stories focus in different ways on autonomy as the right to choose and act according to one's own wishes. However, not everyone wishes to make their own choices. In Story 3 (page 9), a pregnant woman is trying to decide whether or not to terminate her pregnancy. She is distressed and indecisive. Finally, she asks her health visitor, with whom she has an established relationship, to make the decision on her behalf. It is possible to argue that respect for this woman's autonomy should lead the health visitor to make the decision for her: it is what she has requested and, incidentally, the request appears reasonable. The woman knows that she needs a decision to be made but cannot make it herself. Yet, to make a decision on a client's behalf (whether a critical and serious decision or a more trivial one) can also be argued to deny the client's autonomy – their right to make their own choice and to have control. Does a client's voluntary and deliberate surrender of autonomy ('Tell me what to do') put power back in the hands of the professional? And is it then the moral responsibility of the professional to exercise that power?

Since choices cannot be made without information, information-giving is also essential in the provision of individual care. There may be difficulties for the nurse in knowing what and how much information to give and when to give it, and it is also possible that, no matter how clearly and skilfully communicated, information is not understood. But these difficulties do not affect the overriding moral obligation to inform. It is clear, too, that sharing information with the client is an important means of creating greater equality within the nurse-client relationship, and that to withhold information, or misinform, threatens and may destroy an individual's autonomy. Are there, however, circumstances in which withholding information might be justified?

Stories 4, 6 and 7 (pages 10, 13 and 14) all describe situations in which information is withheld. In Story 4, a nurse is asked by the parents of her 19-year-old patient to withhold information about her terminal cancer. The nurse agrees – although reflecting on her decision later, she regrets it. It is clear that the denial of information to the patient also denies her the power to choose whether she should be treated and how she should die. In Story 6, a nurse tranquillises a patient without his knowledge. The nurse himself is clear, in telling this story, that this was indefensible practice, denying the patient his autonomy and rights. In Story 7, a nurse in an A&E department informs the police about a patient who is drunk. When the patient drives away from the hospital after treatment, he is arrested. By not telling the patient that she was going to inform the police, this nurse denied the patient the opportunity to make his own choice about whether to drive or not.

However, these stories also raise questions to do with respect for the autonomy of others beside the patient. Gillon[6] describes respect for autonomy as 'the moral obligation to respect the autonomy of others in so far as such respect is compatible with equal respect for the autonomy of all those potentially affected'. By tranquillising the disruptive patient in Story 6, did the nurse protect the autonomy of others on the ward? The drunk driver in Story 7 was similarly a danger to others. Does this justify the nurse's action? In Story 4, is it possible that the nurse, though denying the autonomy of the patient, acted in support of the patient's parents and enabled them to care for their daughter in the way that they wanted? If so, would this sufficiently justify withholding such vital information from the person it most concerns? On the one hand, it could be argued that informing the patient about her illness against her parents' wishes risks destroying family relationships (and what might be described as the autonomy of the family unit) at a critical and difficult time. On the other hand, informing the patient could help her to be autonomous in relation to her parents, which could be important for her – and maybe ultimately even for them. In practice, a nurse would have to consider (though with scant information) the family relationships involved and attempt to assess the risks of either course of action.

In all these stories, denying information to the patient can be seen to be dishonest as well as disempowering. The stories raise questions about whether dishonesty – or any other less than moral or immoral behaviour – can be justified. Story 10 (page 26), which is also about dishonesty, offers a slightly different perspective. Here, a health visitor is concerned about a baby's development. The baby's mother has herself noticed that the baby is slow to sit up and asks the health visitor about it. The health visitor, despite her own anxieties about the baby, reassures the mother by telling her that there is nothing to worry about. She wants to save the mother anxiety that she feels may be unfounded. In contrast to Stories 4, 6 and 7, the health visitor deliberately lies in order, as she thinks, to benefit her client. Her intentions are entirely beneficent, but her statement that there is nothing to worry about is dishonest and misleading. Can such dishonesty – and denial of autonomy – be justified by the intended benefit to the client?

II The nurse–patient/client relationship

Story 8 Questions of trust and judgement

'I was on nights and a woman came in who'd been beaten up by her husband. She was very upset and very, very scared that this guy was going to come looking for her. She wanted to get home because she said that if he didn't see her soon, he'd think she was with somebody else, even though he'd beaten her up and she'd gone to Casualty for treatment. Well, he'd pushed her through a glass window, and she had some quite bad cuts. I said, "Surely in the state you're in, he'd believe that you were in a hospital." But she said, no.

'What this woman needed was a lot of talking to, a lot of confidence-building, before she'd even let us come near her with a needle. And it took about an hour before I'd gained her confidence enough to be able to attend to her wounds. Then we got into the problem of where she was going to go. I didn't think it was a good idea for her to go home. So I suggested I might phone the police. But she said no, because although they might lock her husband up for the night, they'd let him out in the morning, and then he'd beat her up even worse tomorrow.

'Anyway, I talked to this woman for several hours. It turned out she had a mother living not too far away. She didn't want her mother to know what was happening. Apparently, she'd never let on in the three or four years she'd been married that she'd been assaulted by her husband. She'd always covered it up. And she didn't want her mother to know because her mother was quite poorly. I said, I think the time has come now when you've got to tell someone about your problems, because you can't go on like this. And she agreed she would talk to her mother.

'So we needed to get to a phone. And the only phone where there's any privacy is in the office. So we were in there and I got hold of the mother and I got hold of someone who would come and pick this lady up and take her to her mother's house. But then this lady became . . . over-grateful and she put her arms round me and gave me a cuddle. At first I thought it was just her way of showing me some affection after what I'd done because I did feel I'd done quite a lot. I'd done maybe three hours' work for this lady. But then I could see I had got to get out of that room. So how do you do it? You can destroy three hours' good work just like that if you do or say the wrong thing. But at the end of the day the other thing that was in my mind was, I'm a bloke, in this room, on my own with this woman, there's nobody else around and this woman could say anything about me. I don't know her, I *felt* I knew her having talked to her for three hours, but all of a sudden you can wake up and realise you know nothing about this person whatsoever.

'I sat her down and I said, "I think really you know you have to realise where you are and I'm a nurse and I have got other people to see and now we've sorted your problem out I think you just need to get control of your emotions a little bit." I didn't say, "Pull yourself together" but some words a bit like that! I was feeling very worried and I thought, "Is everything she's said true? What sort of stories has she been telling me?" But I do believe she was telling the truth. She was very sincere, very sensible, initially very frightened. It took a long time for her to say anything, and I think what she was saying was the truth.'

Discussion points

- The nurse worked hard to create a relationship with this patient in order to be able to help her. Nevertheless, did he exceed his responsibilities? How much is emotional care a legitimate and necessary part of a nurse's job?

- How do you decide whether to believe/trust a patient? How do you encourage a patient to trust you?

- How could the nurse have protected himself but still helped his patient?

Story 9 What did she want?

'I looked after a woman recently all through her pregnancy. She was someone who had very clear ideas about what she wanted, very clear ideas about wanting to have her baby at home, and very, very definitely not wanting an epidural. That was absolutely not on the agenda. We discussed it carefully and I said to her, "Well, it looks extremely likely that you can get through your labour without an epidural", and I explained what it might mean and said that I would certainly back her in her wishes. But we also looked at the outside chance that if her labour didn't go as she hoped then an epidural might be the best option. And even though she trusted me, because we'd known each other a long time, she wrote all this down, giving clear instructions about what she did and definitely didn't want.

'So she went into labour and she laboured for a time at home. But then the labour wasn't going very well, there was meconium in the waters, and we made a decision to transfer to hospital. We arrived at the hospital, and immediately there was pressure from the medical staff for intervention, and that included an epidural.

'Well, I really felt strongly that my role was to help her to get through without an epidural because I knew from before that she definitely didn't want one. But she was in the very late stages of labour and she was begging me, "I know I said I didn't want one, but now I do." And that's a very difficult situation to find yourself in as a midwife. The doctors told me I was cruel and asked me what I was doing. I showed them the paper, and they said, "But that's neither here nor there." And I said, "I disagree with you, and one of the reasons I disagree with you is that I know I'm going to have to look after this woman for the next 28 days and I'm going to have to live with what we decide now." And she was saying, "I want an epidural now", and I was thinking, "We've only got one centimetre to go, then she'll be fine."

'My decision was to help her through by sitting with her and talking her through the contractions, just helping her get there. After an hour or so she got to the point when she didn't want an epidural any more and she pushed her baby out and she was fine.

'Afterwards I said to her, "Okay, what was that all about then?" And she said "Oh, I know I was saying I wanted an epidural but I didn't really, of course I didn't." Now I knew that she didn't want an epidural. Or at least, I thought I knew. I hoped I knew.'

Discussion points

- What role did clinical experience and professional judgement play in the midwife's decision not to give the epidural? What other factors may have influenced her decision?

- What might your feelings have been as the client in this story?

- In the relationship between a midwife or nurse and a client, are there responsibilities on both sides? What, if any, do you consider are the responsibilities of the client?

- How well can a midwife/nurse know a client or patient?

- Do you feel that the client's gratitude justifies the midwife's decision?

Story 10 'I didn't want to worry her'

'I've been looking after this mother since taking over from her midwife so I've known her a little while and I know she worries a lot about the baby. She's very perceptive, and the fact is, I'm worried too. But I feel that if I tell her so, it will just add to her anxieties. The babe doesn't sleep much at the moment, so she's quite tired and low anyway.

'She came in last week, and I looked at the baby and talked to her. He's not sitting up yet, and for the first time last week she actually said to me, "Surely he should be sitting up by himself by now?" And I didn't really say yes or no but just talked to her generally for a bit, but she came back to it and questioned me quite directly. She said, "I'm really worried. Shouldn't he be sitting up?" And I just felt that I needed a bit longer before I could be really sure that there was a problem and that if I expressed my own worries just then she would have another fortnight or month of dreadful anxiety that might be needless. So I said quite firmly that I didn't feel there was any need to worry.'

Discussion points

● Do you feel the health visitor's response was justifiable? On what grounds?

● What does the health visitor's decision not to share her concern mean for her relationship with this client?

● How do you think the health visitor's decision not to express her own anxieties might affect her relationship with this mother in the future?

Story 11 A sense of betrayal

'When I visited the family that day, the father, Michael, was out but the mother, Jean, and the little girl were both there, and we were able to sit together and have quite a long talk. I was desperately sorry for Jean. She'd been quite badly knocked about by Michael about a year before. I'd tried to support her then, and we'd become quite close. I felt we were friends, really. I certainly felt she would turn to me if things were bad. But until then, so far as I knew, Michael had never touched the children, and over the past few months I'd felt that things had improved a bit.

'But it was while we were talking that I noticed that the little girl was definitely bruised. In fact, Jean wasn't making any attempt to hide it, which she easily could have done. So after a while, I asked her about it. And Jean said that yes, it had been Michael, and that she was worried. She wanted to talk to me, but she asked me not to go to the social services. She said she and Michael had talked about it and he'd promised it wouldn't happen again . . . She said several times, "You won't tell, will you?"

'I was trying to weigh up whether it would be best to try to keep close to Jean and keep the relationship going with her, or whether I should talk to the social workers. And I really found that very difficult. But in the end I felt it would be most helpful just at that time if I could keep the relationship going with Jean and if she felt she could really trust me. So I promised that I wouldn't report it.

'And then I got outside, and it all looked quite different, and I knew I just couldn't take the risk. So I went to the social services straightaway.'

Discussion points

- What factors would you consider in trying to decide whether or not to report a case like this?

- The health visitor describes her feelings about her relationship with Jean. What might Jean's feelings be? How do you think these feelings might be changed by the health visitor reporting her child's bruising?

- What might the consequences have been if the health visitor had not mentioned the bruising to the mother at all and had gone straight to the social services?

● How might the health visitor have kept Jean's trust but still reported the child's bruising?

Commentary: The nurse-patient/client relationship

Something has already been said about the inequalities inherent in the relationship between people who give care and people who need and receive it, and about the difficulties that these inequalities may create in caring for clients as people. It has been suggested that a more equal and collaborative relationship can be created by giving choice, information and power to the client. For the nurse's part, this will almost certainly involve the surrender of some professional power and the acceptance of some risk, although it is important to note that some patients may *choose* a non-participative or less powerful role.

However, it is not only the unequal power relations between nurses and clients that make caring for clients as people difficult. Efforts to provide individual and holistic care – to care for the whole person – may dramatically alter the nurse–client relationship and may give rise to some uncertainty and confusion about the nature of the relationship itself. This too may lead to difficulty.

If a nurse's task is considered to be to attend solely to a client's physical needs (and in some cases it may be so), the nurse–client relationship will be relatively remote. Despite the closeness often created by giving physical care, the relationship may remain quite impersonal and possibly little more than the relationship between a provider and a consumer of a service. But if a nurse is to provide holistic care, he or she must not only attend to the client's physical needs but also take account of his or her emotional, psychological or spiritual needs, adapting the care that is given accordingly. Furthermore, this must be done individually for each client. This kind of care both implies and demands a closer and more complicated relationship and requires that the nurse knows at least something, if not a great deal, about the client as a person.

In reality, a nurse knows very little about a client as a person, although it is easy to lose sight of this. Within health care, relationships develop rapidly and are intimate almost from the start. The intimacy is artificial, a product of the experience of neediness and care, but it may nonetheless be felt as real by both nurse and client. Both, after all, have reasons which may lead them to consider their relationship to be closer, or more empathic, than it is. From the nurse's point of view, a sense of being close to and understanding the client may make it easier as well as more satisfying to give care. The client, who is likely to be in a dependent role, has an investment in a nurse's understanding, benevolence and reliability.

In Story 8 (page 23), a male nurse working in an A&E department treats a woman who has been pushed through a window by her husband. The woman is upset and frightened. The nurse attends to her wounds and tries to comfort her. In fact, because of her emotional state, he cannot begin to treat her until he has talked to her, established a relationship and built up some trust. This leads him into spending considerable time with the woman, and he helps her to make some arrangements for her safety after she leaves hospital. He is, in the best sense, trying to care for her as a whole person.

The woman then hugs him – he believes in gratitude. Then it seems that the hug is meant to mean more. He wonders whether he has misjudged her. Has she been lying to him? Has she led him on? In caring for her, he has made a series of judgements based on his 'knowledge' of her and his assessment of her needs. Now he realises that these judgements had only a flimsy basis and could have been mistaken. Reflecting on the incident later, he does not consider that he should have behaved differently but is conscious of the risks involved in creating this kind of caring relationship.

The story highlights the limitations of the nurse–client relationship – a relationship based on limited personal knowledge, constructed not as a matter of choice but for certain purposes and within certain, often unconducive circumstances. Caring for the client as a person demands human interaction, and people should be cared for with humanity. But clearly human interaction within the nurse–client relationship will always be constrained, and awareness of what is not and can never be known about a client is as vital in individualised care as the sensitive use of what is known.

Story 9 (page 25), however, seems to suggest that a nurse's knowledge of her client is not only reliable but also a useful clinical tool. Here the relationship has developed over a period of months. The midwife who tells the story has cared for the woman from the start of her pregnancy. They have had opportunities to talk together about what the woman wants when she is in labour, and the woman has stated clearly that she does not want an epidural. So, when the woman is in the late stages of labour and asks urgently for an epidural, the midwife feels secure and confident enough in her relationship with her client to refuse.

Unlike the relationship in Story 8, the midwife-client relationship has developed (and has been developed) gradually over a lengthy period of time. As a result, the midwife feels that she has a good understanding of what her client wants. But while a positive, established relationship with a client may lessen the risk of misjudging his or her wishes and needs, it cannot obviate that risk. For this midwife, it merely enabled her to predict with greater confidence the likely consequence of her decision – namely, that her client would later be pleased not to have had the epidural. In this particular case, her prediction proved correct.

However, it can also be argued, since consequences in situations of this kind can rarely if ever be predicted with certainty, that the midwife's duty was to meet the woman's request, even though it contradicted her earlier plans for managing her labour. Using this approach, whatever the midwife's feelings about the possible consequences of her action, she would nevertheless have felt that her duty to meet her client's request was more important, and would therefore have given the epidural. Some may feel that this course of action is in fact the less risky: it can at least be understood and agreed by both sides in advance. Both possible courses of action need to be considered not only from the midwife's but also the pregnant woman's point of view, considering in both cases the implications for the midwife-client relationship.

In Story 9, in attempting to predict the likely consequence of a decision not to give an epidural, the midwife is using not only what she believes she knows about her client as a person but also her own clinical experience. She has seen many women in late first-stage labour and in her experience it is not unusual for them to say things they do not mean. However, although experience plays a valuable and sometimes vital role in all professional judgements, it is also important to consider the implications of this way of working for the exceptional woman who means what she says and wants what she asks for. While it may be unusual, in the midwife's experience, for women to mean what they say at this particular stage in labour, and usual for them to ask for what they do not really want, the use of such experience in practice is likely to jeopardise the interests of women (no matter how few) who do not fit the pattern. What, then, does this mean for individualised care?

Story 10 (page 26) offers an interesting comparison. Here too, a professional makes a decision based on prediction of consequences. Knowing a mother to be worried about her baby's development, a health visitor chooses to reassure her, even though she is herself worried. She feels this will prevent the mother continuing to worry, and intends to tell the mother the truth when she herself becomes certain that there is genuine cause for concern. Although the health visitor predicts a short-term benefit for the mother, it is clear that her decision could also have long-term consequences for her relationship with her client, and it is interesting to consider what her decision says about, and means for, her present relationship with that client. In an equal relationship between nurse and client, both partners have rights and responsibilities. However, it may be difficult if not impossible for the client to take responsibility and exercise power within the relationship if he or she cannot absolutely trust and depend on the nurse's honesty and openness.

Story 11 (page 27) is also about trust and the way in which trust is created and maintained within the nurse–client relationship. The health visitor in this story has worked to create a trusting relationship with a woman whose husband is violent. She feels this relationship is the key to giving the woman the support and care she needs. So, on finding that the father has (as the mother confirms) hurt one of the children, the health visitor at first agrees to the mother's request not to report the incident. Later, she changes her mind and goes to the social services, although she does not tell the mother she is doing so.

The health visitor feels that she has betrayed the mother's trust. The mother had asked her not to report the incident, and yet the health visitor had done so. Although her duty to protect the child may be considered beyond dispute, (few would question her eventual decision), she feels nevertheless that doing her duty may have negative consequences for her relationship with her client and perhaps may even limit her ability to support the family and protect the child in the future.

While this may be true, it is arguable that the betrayal of trust consists not so much in her decision to report the bruising but in her failure to tell the mother that she was going to do so. What could be her reasons for withholding this information? And what does this suggest about her understanding of her relationship with her client and her own obligations within it?

Although the health visitor in this story feels that her relationship with her client is akin to friendship, it is in fact constrained by her professional role and, in this case, by her duty to protect the child. It is important to recognise and identify the ways in which professional obligations (or even tasks) will influence and define the nurse–client relationship, and to consider how a positive relationship can be built, across personal, cultural or other difference, with some understanding on both sides of the real and often necessary limitations.

Story 12 Taking sides

'I remember a 14-year-old girl who was brought to A&E because she'd been kicked in the stomach at school. She was brought in by her school teacher and when we were alone she told me she was about six weeks' pregnant. She hadn't told anyone; she hadn't told her mum.

'So her mum arrived and I had to treat this girl. But she didn't want me to tell her mum she was pregnant. I said, "Have you discussed this with your mum?" And she said, "No, she'll kill me, I don't want her to know."

'This girl was 14, she was a sensible girl, she knew what she was doing. So I accepted her decision, I took her side. So I'm taking this girl for a scan and of course I can't tell the mum why. And the mum said, "Why is she going for a scan?" And I was stuck really in the middle and I said, "We're just taking her for a scan to see if any damage has been done." It wasn't exactly a lie because she'd been kicked in the abdomen, but I found it really traumatic.

'It wasn't difficult to decide to take the girl's side, but it was difficult not telling the mother. It was very difficult keeping my promise.'

Discussion points

- What are the arguments to support the nurse's decision to take the girl's side?

- What are the arguments in favour of telling the mother about her daughter's pregnancy?

- What is the nurse's responsibility in this situation?

Story 13 For whose good?

'An elderly lady with dementia came to us for assessment. I was her primary nurse. And she was telling me explicitly and very clearly that she wanted to go home.

'She lived with her son, and her son seemed to be under a great deal of stress looking after her. He was suffering from depression and panic attacks and stress-related illnesses. He was taking time off work sick, and it was obviously connected with how he felt about looking after his mother and the burden of caring for her 24 hours a day.

'And it's difficult, because on the one hand you are the patient's advocate and you say, 'This woman wants to go home. She doesn't want to be in residential care'. But then you also have the son coming to you and crying and saying, "I just won't be able to cope with her at home." And both the GP and the consultant recognised that it would be detrimental to the son's mental health for her to go home, yet it would be detrimental to the mother's mental well-being and personhood for her to be ignored and forced to go into a residential home.

'We talked to the son, and he was very upset because he didn't want to cause his mother further distress but at the same time he was clearly saying she couldn't go home. So it was kind of passed over. It was agreed that she couldn't go home until he was better, so in the meantime she went to a continuing care ward.'

Discussion points

- What is the role of the primary nurse in this situation? How can she best support her patient?

- What responsibility, if any, does the nurse have towards the son?

- Are there occasions when the needs of a patient's family could be considered more important than the patient's needs?

Story 14 'We thought we knew best'

'Steve had been on my ward for months. He'd had quite a severe stroke, and then at least two more, and he was left unsteady on his feet and he couldn't swallow and needed feeding by tube. He could just about use all his limbs, but not in any refined way, so caring for himself was very difficult. He couldn't speak but he could show us what he liked and didn't like and whether he approved or disapproved. The major effect he seemed to have been left with was a form of dementia, and he just couldn't function as he'd previously done. Sometimes his behaviour was very inappropriate. He'd take a swing at you if he didn't like the look of you, or go to the toilet wherever he happened to be, or expose himself.

'Anyway, we spent a lot of time trying to understand how he wanted things and how he liked things doing. And caring for him within the hospital setting like that made us feel that the likelihood of him being able to manage in the community was remote.

'He had two grown-up daughters and a son. His wife had died when the children were quite young, and he'd brought them up on his own, so the children felt tremendously loyal towards him and they loved him and wanted him home and wanted to look after him. The trouble was that that wasn't backed up by what we saw when they came to visit. We'd say, "Why don't you take Steve for a walk round the hospital?" And they'd take him out and would find it very difficult to handle and then they wouldn't come in for days on end. So we couldn't see how they could look after him if they took him home. They said they wanted it, but we just couldn't see it happening. The oldest daughter was in her mid-twenties and had two young children and a job, and the other two were young and were busy enjoying life.

'So in the end we arranged for him to go to a nursing home, even though the family were saying they really did want to look after him themselves. We talked with them and in the end they agreed that it was a reasonable decision and they went along with it and felt okay about it.

37

'Well, Steve arrived in the nursing home and soon afterwards he took matters into his own hands and walked out! And he ended up being discharged home. And now he lives in a suburb, and all the bus drivers there know not to let him on the bus, and he wanders round his little bit of the town, and people know him and ultimately the outcome has been a good one.

'We thought we knew best and we had the best of intentions, but we didn't stretch ourselves beyond what we thought was safe. And even though Steve and his family didn't really suffer that much, I feel quite bad that we didn't have the courage to take the risk ... In the end their resources proved bigger than our imagination.'

Discussion points

- Was it justifiable to persuade the family to accept a decision they did not want? On what grounds?

- What is your assessment of the risk of sending Steve home to live with his family? What might the consequences have been?

- Are there occasions when the needs of a patient's family could be considered more important than the patient's needs?

Story 15 Whose advocate?

'We have one long-term patient who's been here for six months. She's unconscious and doesn't communicate. No one, including the consultant neurologist, is absolutely sure what is wrong with her.

'She developed a series of infections, and I asked the medical staff whether we could send some specimens off to the laboratory. They were quite shocked and said, no, they didn't want to send off any specimens because that would mean they would get an answer and then they'd have to treat the patient. The fact is, they didn't want to treat her.

'But I knew that the patient's husband would want her to be treated, and that put me in a very difficult situation. So I made that known to the medical staff and I said I would have to be very honest with the husband if he asked me.

'But thinking about it further, I felt that it was a deception not to raise something with the husband, knowing that it was important to him. So I did speak to him and I told him that she had these infections and that if he wanted his wife to be treated, he needed to insist to the medical staff that they treated her.

'The conflict occurs because if you can't ask the patient (and in this case we couldn't), then you ask the relatives as an indicator of the patient's values. If the relatives agree with what the medical team want to do then there's no problem. But if they disagree, it is very problematic.'

Discussion points

- As the patient's advocate, should the nurse take the side of the patient or family, even, if necessary, in opposition to medical staff?

- How can a nurse best fulfil his or her role as the patient's advocate if the patient is unable to communicate? Is it acceptable to use a relative or friend of the patient as 'an indicator of the patient's values'? What are the risks involved in doing this?

- In this nurse's place, how would you approach the husband and what would you wish to discuss with him?

Commentary: The nurse–family relationship

Relatives and friends may sometimes be involved in a client's care. If, for example, a client is unable to communicate, or is a baby or small child, or mentally or physically disabled, family and friends are likely to play a crucial role. The nurse may then have to develop a relationship both with the client (in so far as that is possible) and the client's family or friends. Sometimes the relationship with the client may be so limited that the nurse-family relationship must substitute for it.

Ideally, nurse, family, friends and client all work together in these circumstances. But it is not unusual for the needs or wishes of relatives, and the needs or wishes of a client, to be in conflict. It may then become very difficult to reach ethical decisions about a client's care, and for the professionals concerned there are likely to be questions of – or feelings about – loyalty.

Story 13 (page 36) illustrates this dilemma. An elderly woman with dementia wishes to be discharged from hospital. She wants to go home, not into residential care. But her son, who looks after her at home, is ill and worn down by the job of caring for her and says he cannot cope. Should the elderly woman be sent to a residential home against her wishes?

This is a stark story. Unless extensive community support can be arranged, there can be no satisfactory answer which will accommodate the needs of both mother and son. A pragmatic decision is therefore made to send the mother to a continuing care ward – at least until her son is better and able to care for her. The nurse involved felt unhappy about this solution. Had she let her patient down?

Whatever practical solution is decided on in a situation like this, it is important to consider the *process* by which a decision is reached. The nurse cannot be reassured that the decision was a good one for her patient, even though it may have been the best possible in the circumstances, but she can and should feel assured that the process by which the decision was reached was rigorous and sound.

This story about the elderly woman and her son can be compared with Story 4 (page 10), in which a 19-year-old girl is not treated for cancer at the request of her parents. Her parents ask that she is not told that her cancer is terminal, nor about the palliative treatment she could receive. Although it may seem clear that it is unethical in this situation for the girl not to be given full information about her illness and so enabled to make her own decision about her treatment, it is also important to reflect on the feelings of the parents and to consider whether or not they may also have some rights in this situation. Similar questions arise about Story 12 (page 35), in which a 14-year-old girl asks a nurse not to tell her mother that she is pregnant. The nurse agrees. But does the girl's mother have any right to know?

These questions can be addressed most usefully not in terms of individual rights but through consideration of the responsibilities of the nurse. The responsibilities of the nurse to the patient are relatively clear – as set down, for example, in the *UKCC Code of Professional Practice.*[7] But does the nurse also have responsibilities towards the patient's family? What, in other words, does the nurse 'owe' the parents of the girl with cancer or the mother of the pregnant schoolgirl?

It is arguable, if a nurse's first allegiance is to the patient, that what is owed to the patient's family is no more than what is necessary, beneficial and right for the patient. But it is important to recognise the sensitive and difficult judgements that may be involved. For example, the nurse caring for the elderly woman with dementia (Story 13) might judge that it would not be in the woman's interests to be sent home to be cared for by someone unable to give good care. The nurse caring for the cancer patient (Story 4) might decide that she should not comply with the parents' request to conceal information from their daughter because this would not be in the interests of the daughter. The nurse caring for the pregnant teenager (Story 12) might consider that it was not in the daughter's interests for her mother to be told about her pregnancy. However, all these judgements are open to debate and demonstrate the potential for paternalism in these and similar situations.

A further question concerns the nurse's role. In Story 12, it could be argued that the mother should know of her daughter's pregnancy. Is it, then, the nurse's job to inform her? Different professionals are likely to hold different opinions about this, and it is important to explore other practical possibilities for supporting both the patient and her family beyond the simple question of 'telling or not'.

The nurse's dilemma in Story 15 (page 38) is very different. A woman who has been in intensive care for six months has developed an infection. She cannot communicate. Doctors in the team refuse to investigate the infection because they do not feel it is appropriate to treat the patient. The nurse involved, however, knows that the woman's husband would want her to be treated and therefore decides to speak to the husband and encourage him to speak to the doctors.

The nurse's difficulty is two-fold. First, there is disagreement within the team. She feels that the infection should be investigated, the medical staff do not. Second, this disagreement is difficult to resolve because the patient herself cannot speak. The wishes of the husband are the only available guide to the likely wishes of the patient (or may, perhaps, be considered as important in their own right).

Even if there is evidence that the relationship between the husband and wife is close and that the husband is therefore likely to know what his wife would want, the situation is still clearly risky. If a nurse feels that the views and wishes of family or friends are not reliable or are even wrong, then the risk is plain. Suppose, in a similar situation, a family asks that their unconscious relative continues to receive unpleasant and painful treatment, even though this is medically inappropriate? Suppose the patient cannot communicate, and there is conflict in the family about what care should be given? Whose views should be followed?

Story 14 (page 37) illustrates this dilemma. Steve is severely disabled by a stroke and needs care. The nurses, who have cared for him over a lengthy period of time and feel they know his needs well, consider that his family will not be able to look after him. His three children want to look after him at home but they are persuaded by the nursing team that Steve should be sent to a nursing home. He makes a rapid escape and is subsequently discharged home where his family look after him as they had originally wished to do.

The nurse who tells this story comments that he and others in his team felt unable to take the risk involved in sending Steve home. This is later (with the benefit of hindsight) a matter of regret. Whatever the outcome for Steve, was it legitimate to disregard the wishes of the family in (as it was thought) Steve's best interests?

When a patient is very dependent, the development of a positive, working relationship with family or friends is likely to be particularly important. In some situations, this relationship will become a substitute – at least temporarily – for the direct nurse-client relationship. But a relationship with relatives or friends will inevitably be very different, and the nurse must be cautious in interpreting the views and wishes of those connected with the patient, no matter how close their connections.

IV The role and responsibilities of the nurse

Story 16 Breaking bad news

'A youngish man, mid-40s, died suddenly and I had to break the news to his wife. She was only about 35. The fact they were so young seemed to make it worse.

'I came into the room and she was on her own, and I sat down and said, "I'm very sorry but I'm afraid your husband has died." And I was just preparing myself to say the things that you usually say, you know, "I'm sorry but there was nothing else we could do, we did our best", and so on, and she just sat there and I was waiting for this flood of tears and a reaction, and it didn't happen. She said very calmly, "Thank God for that."

'Well, I just didn't know what to do. I was quite junior at the time. And this woman said, "You must think I'm awful for saying this but that man was the worst man you could ever meet in your life," and she started to tell me about some of the things he had done. It was horrible, hearing this about a man when we'd just spent 20 minutes trying our best to save his life.

'She said, "The thing is, his mother hates me. He could never do anything wrong in her eyes, and everything was always my fault. And the first thing she'll want to know when she comes to the hospital is, am I grieving? But I can't grieve, because I'm glad he's dead.' And she said, 'I don't want you tell her I'm here and I don't want her to know how I feel. I want her to know that I'm upset because it will make life a lot easier later."

'Well, lo and behold, the mother arrived 20 seconds later, and I took her to another room and said the same thing, that her son had died. And straightaway, just like the daughter had said she would, she wanted to know whether her daughter-in-law was in the hospital and whether she was grieving. So I thought to myself, I'm going to lie, because I liked this woman, the daughter-in-law, and to me she seemed sincere. So I lied and I said to the mother, "Your daughter-in-law's gone home very upset." And I thought, well what else can I do? Because the last thing I wanted was for this woman to meet her daughter-in-law and start an argument, because I didn't know how I would handle it.

'So there I am going backwards and forwards between these two ladies, lying to one and more or less telling the truth to the other but telling it her way, the way she wanted. And eventually I got rid of – well, that sounds of awful, but that's how it seemed – I got rid of them both separately.

'The point is, I made my decision that I was going to stand by the wife of this man because I believed her. And it was just intuition, and I don't know whether she was right or whether she was wrong. But the woman seemed to have a warmth about her and the mother seemed quite cold, and I responded to that and right or wrong I stuck by it.'

Discussion points

- The nurse made a decision based on intuition. What were the risks involved?

- Do you feel it is acceptable to use intuition in this way?

- Do you feel it was the nurse's responsibility to help the wife in the way he did?

- Can you devise any alternative strategies for handling this situation?

Story 17 A vulnerable client

'A community nurse in our team supports a woman who has a mild learning disability. She's about 50 and lives on her own. Her father used to live with her but he died about a year or so ago, and since then she's been quite isolated. She misses him, and we're trying to help her become more socially integrated.

'One thing she's started to do is go to an evening bingo session, and because there aren't any buses, the community nurse has helped her arrange a taxi. Well, the same taxi driver picks her up each week and takes her home at the end of the session, and a relationship has started up between the two of them. It's really the first kind of relationship the woman has ever had.

'At first, the friendship was just platonic but now it seems the taxi driver wants something more physical. The woman is clear about her own sexuality and about what she does and doesn't want from the relationship, and she says that she doesn't want to have sex before she's married.

'The woman is obviously quite vulnerable. She lives alone, the taxi driver knows where she lives, and he's been making rather suggestive phone calls. The woman isn't happy about the phone calls and she's told him to stop, but at the same time she doesn't want the relationship to end.'

Discussion points

- Do you think that someone with a mild learning disability has the same right to the same degree of autonomy as someone with no disability?

- What do you consider to be the nurse's responsibility in this situation?

- How could the nurse intervene most helpfully?

Story 18 For her good but against her will?

'A woman was admitted to our ward who was diagnosed as having quite severe manic depression. She was about 33, with three young children, and she had a history of really bad self-harm. She'd ended up on a liver unit for about ten months after taking an overdose and she'd nearly died on another occasion as well. I knew this woman quite well from past admissions. She was a lovely woman.

'Anyway, when she was admitted, she was quite rational but I thought she was really very depressed. And she wanted to leave. So I said, "I don't want you to leave because I'm really concerned about you." But she said, "I want to leave." So I had to go through the whole process, talking to her about getting her sectioned. And I got the two doctors up and the social worker. The doctors agreed that she was at risk, although she was saying that she was all right, and the social worker said, "No, she says she's going to stay, so I'm not putting her on a section."

'Well, she was still on the ward and I was still really, really concerned about her. So I took the decision to put her on continuous supervision, which means she had a nurse sitting beside her all the time. I was so worried about her. But it was a very difficult situation for me. It was as though I was saying to her, "We're sitting with you so that you can't leave, and if you try to leave, you'll be sectioned." But she'd been assessed and she hadn't been sectioned. It was very, very difficult.

'As the day went on she got more and more ill and ended up really needing quite a lot of support and lots of medication. In the end, she did have to be sectioned.

'About a month later I talked with her, and she said she was really glad that I'd sat with her because she was going to kill herself. She said she'd lied to the doctors and social worker and had said she was all right.

'I think I decided I didn't want her to die, because I thought that she was mentally ill and it was her mental illness that was making her want to die. I also knew that she really loved her children and they really loved her and I felt that I had to help to keep her alive for her children. Anyway, that's what I decided, and it turned out all right. But I didn't feel it was the right decision at the time, and if I'd decided not to interfere, I wouldn't have felt that was right either.'

Discussion points

- Since the woman was assessed as rational, was it justifiable for the nurse to decide to prevent her from leaving the ward? On what grounds?

- Whose responsibility was it to ensure this woman received the right treatment?

Story 19 Problems of priorities

'You have one patient who is sitting alone and unstimulated in a corner and you have another who has just had diarrhoea on the floor. And the person with the diarrhoea shoots to the top of your list of priorities.

'You might be helping someone who is very dependent to have a meal. Food is the highlight of their day. It's a sensory pleasure and it's real attention and one-to-one contact. And the phone rings. It's almost an automatic response just to drop everything and go to answer the phone.'

Discussion points

- On what basis should priorities for nursing care be decided?

- To what extent can, or should, these priorities be set by the individual practitioner?

- How can you balance the time you give to visible and invisible care?

Story 20 The tea trolley

'Every afternoon the tea trolley will come down the ward, and the man who pushes the trolley asks each patient whether they'd like a cup of tea. And routinely, if he doesn't get an answer, he'll just walk on by. Because he has to get his tea trolley back by a certain time so he can go home on time. So he doesn't want to go to find the nurse to find out whether the patient can have a cup of tea or not. So no cup of tea is left.'

Discussion points

- Identify exactly what is unethical about this situation.

- Whose responsibility is it to rectify this situation?

- What kind of changes are needed? How can they be brought about?

Story 21 If only . . .

'I looked after a woman who was having her first baby. I met her fairly early on in her pregnancy and got to know her well. She had a history of depression and she'd been an in-patient for that. She'd made an attempt at medical training but hadn't completed it because of her mental illness, although it wasn't severe.

'While she was a medical student, her sister had her first baby and afterwards went through a severe puerperal psychosis. She was admitted to hospital and given ECT, and the woman I was looking after was with her. She had been absolutely shocked and devastated and upset by what her sister had gone through. But her sister had recovered and had gone on to have three more children and had been absolutely fine. But my client spent a lot of time during her pregnancy worrying about whether she would have a psychosis because she realised that there could be a connection between her own mental history and the possibility of developing this, plus the fact that her sister had had one. And we talked at length antenatally about what would happen if she did become ill postnatally and we brought in the community psychiatrist who came and saw her at home and talked to her. We made sure there was good support for her after the birth. Her parents were around.

'And she was clear that the best way for her to have her baby would be at home with people she knew and no interference from outsiders. And she had her baby at home, and then six to seven days later she developed an acute psychosis and had to be admitted to hospital and she was admitted to a mother-and-baby unit.

'I went to visit her in the unit and kept in touch with her. And she would ring me at home frequently and say things like, "You won't let them give me ECT, will you? You promise you won't?" And we talked about it and she wasn't stable mentally at all but I just said, "No, I know what you want and I'm not going to push for that at all." And she was treated with drugs.

'But when the baby was three months old and she was still in the psychiatric unit, she gave him his breakfast one morning and then walked out and threw herself under a train and killed herself. And the very first thing I thought was, maybe I could have stopped that. Maybe if I hadn't listened to what she was asking me to do, we would still have her here today. What I did was listen to what she said she wanted all the way along. And it still rests with me now that she could be here today if I as a professional had said, "We need to act here and take these decisions out of her hands, we need to do something"'

Discussion points

- The midwife who told this story felt that the woman did not want to die. Would your thoughts about the story be different if the woman had said that she *did* want to die?

- Is it justifiable to ignore a client's requests if you believe that complying would be harmful to them or to others?

- What was the midwife's responsibility towards her client in this situation?

Commentary: The role and responsibilities of the nurse

Caring for clients as people raises important questions for nurses about their own role and responsibilities, not only in relation to clients but also in relation to professional colleagues and the organisation within which they work. Individual, holistic care inevitably makes demands on the nurse not just as a professional but also as a person, and while it is often suggested that it is desirable for nurses to use their humanity within their professional role, the extent to which this is appropriate and possible, either for the nurse or for the patient, is also questionable. The use of intuition in decision-making about care is a case in point.

In Story 16 (page 43), a nurse in an A&E department faces the task of telling a woman about her husband's death. He breaks the news to her as gently as possible and prepares himself to comfort and help her as best he can. Astonishingly, she is pleased and relieved. She tells the nurse that her husband was 'the worst man you could ever meet'.

The nurse now becomes involved in a complicated family situation. The dead man's mother comes to the hospital. The man's wife explains that her mother-in-law does not like her. She asks the nurse not to tell her mother-in-law that she is in the hospital, and to tell her that she (the wife) is distressed and grieving for her husband.

The nurse agrees to lie on the wife's behalf. He believes her, and decides to take her side. This judgement is, he says, intuitive. He *feels* that the wife is right and the mother-in-law is wrong, and this feeling is strong enough for him to act upon. Later, on reflection, he agrees that he does not and cannot *know* whether his judgement was correct, and certainly it had no rational basis.

Nurses frequently use what might be called intuition in giving care. For example, a nurse may say, on no apparently rational basis, that she *feels* a patient's colour is wrong, or that she *feels* a patient would be helped by being moved into a different position. But these are probably not purely intuitive feelings. They are clinical judgements informed not just by human feeling but also by professional experience. On other occasions, professional experience may be less relevant, as in Story 16. Here the nurse was using intuitive feeling, but not professional experience or expertise.

Intuition is inevitably a risky tool, although sometimes there may be little else available to guide decision-making. Nurses who have used their intuition successfully may justify it on those grounds, but it is possible to imagine situations in which intuitive decisions could be entirely mistaken and damaging. Is it, then, wrong to use it?

All human interaction involves emotion: it is not merely rational. This is as true for professionals in their relationships with clients as it is in other human relationships. All professionals inevitably use, in different ways and to different degrees, personal feelings and experience in their interaction with clients, and caring for clients as people particularly stresses the use of human qualities such as warmth and empathy. However, the use of feeling and intuition, however desirable and potentially beneficial, is also potentially dangerous for the client and needs to be restrained within some rational framework.

Professional ethics, as formulated, for example, in the *UKCC Code of Professional Conduct*[7] and *The Scope of Professional Practice*,[8] provide an essential framework of rules, but these are painted with a broad brush. More helpful, perhaps, in addressing ethical problems in everyday practice, is the framework provided by policy, by agreed principles of good practice, and by a philosophy of care carefully developed and agreed within a health care team.

A different question also raised by Story 16 is whether this nurse was led by his intuitive feeling to act outside the limits of his professional role. Was it or was it not part of his responsibility to lie to the mother-in-law on the wife's behalf? If, on consideration, this seems to fall outside the boundaries of his responsibilities, then it is useful to consider what factors may have led him to act as he did. The principle of individual and personal care involves an extension of responsibility, beyond the patient to the person. But where does this responsibility end? Can it include a responsibility to lie on a patient's behalf?

Story 17 (page 45) describes a developing relationship between a woman with a learning disability and the man who drives her to and from a weekly bingo session. The woman lives independently with support from a community nurse. The woman welcomes the relationship with the taxi driver but wants it to remain platonic. The taxi driver wants more from the relationship and has begun to make suggestive phone calls. The woman is obviously very vulnerable. Is it the responsibility of the nurse to intervene in this situation, and if so, what kind of intervention might be most moral? In Story 18 (page 46), a nurse prevents a woman from committing suicide. The woman has been assessed as rational, but the nurse (using not only intuition but also her professional judgement and experience) feels strongly that she is mentally ill and does not really want to die. Can the nurse's interference be justified?

Both stories demonstrate the difficulties involved in balancing professional responsibility with respect for the autonomy of the client. In both stories, the dilemma consists in deciding whether it is an invasion of the autonomy of the client to intervene, or an abdication of professional responsibility to hold back. And what exactly is the nature of the responsibility involved? If the woman in Story 17 had confided her difficulty to a friend, would the moral responsibility of that friend be different from the responsibility of the community nurse? The difference may perhaps lie in the commitment of the nurse to benefit (and not harm) the client. This is a professional commitment, and professional training is aimed at enabling the nurse to fulfil that commitment. If, then, a decision *not* to act is likely to cause harm to the client (a sin of omission), it is arguably the professional's responsibility to take action. The client may, however, see things very differently and will, if competent and rational, be the best judge of the limits beyond which intervention becomes inappropriate.

It is interesting to compare Story 3 (page 9), in which a woman who cannot decide whether or not to terminate her pregnancy asks her health visitor to advise her. What, in this case, is the health visitor's responsibility? Plainly, she should try to enable the woman to reach her own decision. But what if the woman is unable – and not only unable but unwilling – to make up her mind? Suppose she actually *wants* the health visitor to intervene? Is it then the health visitor's role to advise her? Is this a responsibility that any health care worker can be fairly asked to assume?

Issues to do with role and responsibility inevitably become more complicated when a client is, for whatever reason, especially vulnerable. In Story 21 (page 48), a woman with a history of mental instability suffers a severe puerperal psychosis after the birth of her first baby. She is admitted to a psychiatric unit and asks her midwife, with whom she has a trusting relationship, not to let her be given ECT. She has seen her sister treated in this way for the same condition and despite the successful outcome, is terrified of receiving the same treatment. The midwife, aware of the woman's experiences and perhaps feeling the obligations created by a good and 'close' relationship with this client, assures the woman that she will not be given ECT. When the woman abandons her baby and kills herself, the midwife wonders whether ECT would in fact have been appropriate and whether her own well-intentioned support had in fact denied the woman this option. She feels regretful and confused and wonders whether she should not have listened to her client.

The story is extreme but highlights the difficulties that exist within every nurse-client relationship. The midwife felt a particularly strong obligation towards this woman because she knew her over a long period of time and felt she was a friend. This feeling of friendship, and a sense of knowing and even intuitively understanding the client, may be helpful to caregivers. But it is also important to question whether it was the midwife's responsibility to support her client's wish not to have ECT. Was this outside her area of professional expertise and, since the woman was hospitalised and receiving psychiatric care, outside the limits of her responsibility? Or did her close relationship with her client create obligations that it was her responsibility to fulfil? In considering these questions, it is important to be aware that responsibility, though often burdensome, may also confer power and control.

Frequently, however, responsibilities bring a sense not of power but powerlessness. Stories 7 and 20 (pages 14 and 48), for example, illustrate the day-to-day ethical dilemmas that nurses commonly experience, yet it is not immediately or obviously within their power to address them. What can or should a nurse do to ensure that a patient who cannot ask for a cup of tea still receives one? How should a nurse decide whether to answer the phone or continue to help a very dependent patient to eat a meal? The ethos of the organisations in which nurses work is clearly influential in such situations and may facilitate or hinder the development of ethical practice. In Story 5 (page 12), nurses are able to make a creative change in policy and practice, opening the locked door of a dementia unit and accompanying patients when they wish to go out. Change of this kind is not easily achieved and is unlikely to be achieved at all outside the context of a strong team philosophy of individualised care.

Many other stories can be seen to raise urgent issues about resources. In Story 6, for example, patients are tranquillised without their knowledge or consent. Is this because they are being cared for in the wrong place by too few and overstretched staff? In Story 13, an elderly woman wants to be discharged home but her son is ill and cannot care for her. Could this situation have been resolved if support was available in the community? In Story 15, doctors do not wish to treat a woman in intensive care. Is there an issue here about the use of limited intensive care beds?

Such difficulties, which are managerial and organisational concerns, directly influence and circumscribe the scope of nurses' ethical thinking and practice, and may jeopardise the delivery of individualised care. It is therefore important, in debating ethical issues, to recognise that the individual health care worker can only develop his or her practice within, and with reference to, its context, and that a broader ethical responsibility is also carried by managers and policy-makers.

Chapter 2

Key factors in the development of ethical practice

The following key factors in the development of ethical practice are derived from the stories told in Chapter 1 and by discussion of the problems and uncertainties that the stories record. They are not rules and are intended to be used to focus discussion of ethical issues.

1 Clients should be cared for as individuals, and as people rather than as patients. This means respecting each client as an autonomous person and involves giving clients choice, information and power. Nurses need to understand and be skilled in empowerment.

2 The relationship between nurse and client should, as far as possible, be constructed as an equal relationship. For the nurse, this means treating clients with respect, sharing information, and recognising and facilitating the client's right to make his or her own decisions about treatment and care. It also involves the recognition of the rights and needs of clients who choose not to be informed or participate in their care.

3 Clear, honest and open communication with clients is essential to ethical practice. All nurses need good communication skills, including, importantly, the ability to give information and to listen.

4 Nurses need to develop their own self-awareness. Each nurse brings to his or her interaction with

55

clients experiences, feelings and attitudes which may profoundly influence decisions about care and the way care is given. It is important that nurses have continuing opportunities to examine and reflect upon the way they interact with clients and how their personal moral beliefs and values influence their practice.

5 Individual nurses need to be able to work within a framework of guiding principles and/or a philosophy of care. It is important that these principles are developed, understood and agreed communally and are reviewed and evaluated in relation to everyday practice. It is appropriate and helpful to involve users in the development and/or evaluation of a philosophy of care.

6 All nurses need opportunities to reflect on and discuss their individual practice from an ethical viewpoint. These opportunities may be provided, for example, within clinical supervision. Some group work is essential in order that individual practitioners can develop an awareness of others' experiences and opinions. It is important that users' opinions should also be heard.

7 Ethical thinking and debate should be included in nurses' basic and post-basic training and in in-service training. Some formal and structured learning about ethics is needed to provide a basis of knowledge and understanding.

8 It is essential that work on ethical issues should include consideration of nurses' needs. Recognition and discussion of the rights of clients should also take account of nurses' rights, and work to empower clients should be balanced with work on self-empowerment.

9 Practitioners' experiences of ethical difficulty take place in an organisational context. It is essential that ethical issues are recognised and addressed at an organisational level. This should include the recognition of the moral content and consequences of policies and protocols for both nurses (and other caregivers) and for users.

Chapter 3

Developing work on ethical issues

'Nurses need ethical exploration. That is, they need freely to examine from cases, preferably in their own experience, the conditions which create disparities between what their moral sense tells them and what they are expected to do without question, expected to accept, believe and justify without moral doubt and anxiety.' [9]

Ethical thinking is important for nurses not because it provides clear right or wrong answers to moral dilemmas (for it rarely does so), but because it offers a way of exploring what response might be 'more right', or more accurately, what is 'most moral'. It is an essential tool in decision-making (although it offers no certainty that the decision finally reached is correct), and equally important, it is a means of reflection.

Many of the nurses who related the stories in Chapter 1 had not previously had opportunities to reflect on their experiences from an ethical viewpoint and found it helpful to do so. Formulating and then debating the specifically *moral* questions raised by particular experiences can help nurses develop their awareness of the moral dimension of their everyday practice, their confidence in addressing ethical issues, and their ability to think in ethical terms.

Opportunities to reflect on and discuss experiences of ethical difficulty can be created formally or informally, within a work setting or away from the demands of practice, with other health care workers and/or with people who have little formal knowledge of health care. A wide range of views can help to inform thinking and stimulate and broaden discussion.

Opportunities in practice

Opportunities already exist within practice to facilitate debate around ethical issues. For example, many units in a wide variety of settings hold debriefing meetings to allow the people involved in a particular incident time to talk about what they did, how they felt, and whether the situation could have been handled differently. Similarly, case conferences are held to review progress and explore future plans and may be informed by multi-professional input and a range of different perspectives. Other team meetings and teaching sessions offer similar opportunities for raising ethical concerns.

However, discussions of this kind are often limited to unusual or overtly difficult situations and day-to-day occurrences can be passed over without recognition of their ethical content. It is important to create opportunities to reflect on and discuss the ordinary events of practice, which are frequently ignored because of their ordinariness but which raise significant ethical issues. Clinical supervision, based on reflection and closely related to practice, offers a particularly appropriate means of developing ethical thinking in a more sustained way around everyday events. The supervisee has the opportunity to set the agenda, identifying situations which, however mundane, have been ethically difficult or perplexing, and within supervision there should be time for exploration and debate.

Work in groups

While it is important that ethical thinking is seen as an integral part of practice, practitioners also need opportunities to look at ethical issues in a more focused way. In small discussion groups, participants can learn of others' different approaches and attitudes and test out and review their own ethical stance. To set up and run such groups, it may be appropriate to work with colleagues in training and development units, teaching units in local colleges of education, or specialist groups with an interest in ethics.

Setting up a discussion group

Numbers

Discussion groups must be small if everyone is to be able to participate. Depending on the composition of the group (see below), the experience and familiarity of participants, and the skills of the facilitator, ten to twelve people is probably a maximum. Sometimes it will be important to bring together a whole team, and if this makes a larger group, it will have to be handled differently, probably using two facilitators and doing more work in pairs or small groups which can then be brought back to the group as a whole.

Time and venue

Participants need to have uninterrupted time for their discussion. They should be able to arrive for the beginning of the session and stay until the end, uninterrupted by bleeps, phone calls or other demands on their time. People coming and going during a session are disruptive.

Use a venue that is comfortable and informal, if possible. People need to relax.

Composition of the group

The composition of the group is likely to be determined by its purpose and the proposed content of discussion. If a discussion is to be held around a particular incident, for example, then it is important that everyone (nurses and others) significantly involved in that incident should be present.

It may be important and helpful for the group to be multi-disciplinary (in which case careful thought should be given to an appropriate facilitator). This might mean an inter-professional group involving medical as well as nursing staff, or possibly a group involving, for example, health care assistants, receptionists and other non-nursing team members. Other professional groups, such as social workers or counsellors, work with established ethical codes and their contribution can help to broaden discussion.

Some thought should be given to the difficulty participants may experience in relating their experiences honestly to other members of the group if their line managers, or others to whom they feel responsible, are present.

It may also be very important to include users. A discussion about ethical practice that is not informed by the views of users will lack a crucial dimension. If a decision is taken *not* to include users (and there are reasons why this may be considered best), then it will be important to raise awareness of the limitations of the discussion within the group and, possibly, explore other ways of obtaining users' views. See 'Involving users', below.

Making a contract/ground rules

It is likely that participants will be talking in the group about experiences that are revealing about themselves and clients. It is essential to agree some ground rules for working together at the beginning of the session, and if more sessions follow, the ground rules need to be reiterated and their acceptance agreed with everyone present.

Ground rules should include:

- confidentiality (an agreement not to repeat what is heard outside the group)
- respect for each other (involving listening to each other without interrupting, giving everyone a chance to speak, and not criticising, condemning or insulting other participants)
- speaking for oneself (and not for other people either within the group or outside it)
- the right to opt out. (This should be carefully negotiated. No participant should feel constrained to take part if they feel they cannot or should not do so. Yet all participants should also make some commitment to the group and its purpose.)

Other ground rules may be suggested that are appropriate to the group or its purpose. Ground rules should be discussed, negotiated and agreed within the group. It is legitimate for either participants or the facilitator to refer back to the groundrules, if necessary, as the discussion develops.

Facilitating the group

Good facilitation by an appropriate person who is acceptable to the group is essential.

It is important to consider the relationship between the facilitator and group members. If there is an existing relationship outside the group (for example, the facilitator is a colleague/team member), that relationship may be helpful (in that he or she is known and respected) or, sometimes, a hindrance (if he or she has a managerial role, for example). It may sometimes be appropriate to use an outside facilitator.

The facilitator will need both good groupwork skills and also some knowledge of health care ethics. Discussion that is structured around participants' experiences can easily become rambling and unfocused. It is important that the facilitator is able to keep discussion on track and maintain the ethical viewpoint.

Some experiential exercises may help to prompt discussion and move it on (see 'Exercises', page 67). It is helpful if the facilitator has some experience of working in this way.

The aim and content of discussion

It is important that the specific aim and purpose of the discussion group are clearly established and understood by everyone who takes part. The content and development of the discussion, perhaps along with other activities, should then be consistent with this aim.

For example, a session might be held on truth-telling. The session might be described beforehand as an exploration of the responsibility of caregivers to tell the truth, the aim being to help participants examine their own views and attitudes and develop ideas about ethical practice. Participants could be invited to bring relevant stories about occasions when they found it difficult to tell the truth, or when they lied. Key questions could be discussed in relation to each story. For example:

- Why was it difficult to tell the truth in this situation?
- Was it the caregiver's responsibility to tell the truth?
- What was there to gain, and who gained, from the truth?
- What was there to gain, and who gained, from the truth being withheld or a lie?

- Can the group agree any general principle(s) about truth-telling?
- If a story concerns lying, can the group think of ways to avoid lying in that particular situation?

If participants are asked to select stories from their practice for discussion in the group, they will need some guidance about the kind of story to bring and how long it should be. It is usually helpful if they have written their story down and reflected upon it beforehand so that they can describe it clearly and articulate their own difficulties and concerns.

Alternatively, it may be preferable to use an imaginary story. This can sometimes give the facilitator more control and make it easier to focus discussion. A story made up or borrowed by the facilitator can be circulated to participants beforehand, along with questions for them to consider. In this way, participants can prepare themselves for discussion which may then be more productive. Stories from Chapter 1 may be used in this way.

Involving users

It is arguable that the involvement of users in discussions on health care ethics is not desirable but essential. It cannot be considered ethical for users' experiences and needs to be represented by professionals; nor for professionals' ideas to go unchallenged by those for whom they care. However, there are drawbacks and difficulties in setting up discussion groups involving users, and if this is attempted, it must be done with care.

It is inappropriate to invite users to discuss issues arising from their own care: if problems have been experienced, a discussion group is not an appropriate forum in which to air them. On the other hand, many users will find it difficult to discuss health care issues in general terms and put forward and maintain the user's point of view. Some careful thought therefore needs to be given to whom to invite to participate. Users who are already involved in collaborative work with professionals (for example, on community health councils, maternity services liaison committees or through voluntary groups), or those working in advocacy or as linkworkers, may be able to take on a representative role.

Any user is in a vulnerable position within a group of professionals. Equal numbers of users and professionals may be difficult to achieve, but there should always be more than one user involved. This is supportive for the users who take part and is likely to bring about a more balanced debate. Like professionals, users do not always agree, and it is important to hear different viewpoints. Users will need to be informed about the purpose and content of the discussion and given time to discuss this, and their role, beforehand.

Professionals, too, are vulnerable. It may be that professionals will feel inhibited by the presence of users, even if they have not been directly involved in their care, and may find it difficult to speak honestly about experiences which have caused them difficulty and maybe even distress. This may jeopardise the discussion to the point where it is considered better for users not to participate. It may, perhaps, be possible to arrange a series of, say, three or four discussion sessions on a developing theme, inviting users to participate in one or two sessions only.

Structuring discussion

The stories in Chapter 1 and others like them can provoke a wide variety of responses. In order to consider the stories in as coherent and progressive a way as possible, it may be helpful to approach them in a structured way. The following approaches are suggestions.

Instant responses

Most people will have some kind of instant response to a story. It can be useful to record this response, either as a starting point for discussion or perhaps in order to be able to set it aside.

Sometimes the way people initially feel when they read a story (irritated or critical, for example) needs to be acknowledged but then put on one side so that they can develop some more objective thinking. People may find it useful to refer back to their immediate reaction later and reconsider it.

Some people may respond to a story simply as a problem to be solved and may make an instant decision about what they themselves would do in the situation described. This too can be recorded before the dilemma is explored more thoroughly.

When registering an immediate response, it is important to do it quickly. This is simply recording a 'gut reaction'.

Some instant responses might include:

'I just felt there was no way out.'
'I wouldn't have lied.'
'That nurse must have felt very sad.'
'I think you have to lie sometimes.'
'What if everyone did that?'
'If I'd been that patient, I'd have been furious.'

What are the issues?

It can sometimes be difficult to move outside a story and consider it objectively. Often people become caught up in the details (of a client's condition or circumstances, for example), whether these are provided by the story or not, and find it hard to identify the ethical issues.

It can be helpful to try to decide, from an ethical viewpoint, what a story is essentially about. Is it, for example, about autonomy? Or power? Or the role of the nurse? What should be the agenda for discussion?

Different people are likely to think differently and this can provide a starting point for debate with each person, or small group of people, explaining their analysis.

Exploring options

Each story provides material for thinking broadly and creatively about how to handle the dilemma that is presented. It is important for everyone to look at as many different options as possible and to consider and articulate carefully all the pros and cons.

In a small group, participants can be asked to brainstorm as many options as possible. This needs to be done freely, making no attempt at this stage to decide what the best option might be.

Participants can then be given time to consider these options and make their own choices, giving their reasons.

What if . . .

In order to think imaginatively about a dilemma and explore it thoroughly, it can be helpful to reconsider it with certain elements changed or added.

In Story 9 (page 25), for example, a midwife decides not to meet a woman's request for an epidural. She says that afterwards the woman is grateful. What if the woman had not been grateful but angry?

In Story 12 (page 35), a 14-year-old girl asks a nurse not to tell her mother that she is pregnant. What if she had asked the nurse to tell her mother? What if the girl had been not 14 but 17 years old? What if the mother had asked the nurse directly whether her daughter was pregnant?

In Story 4 (page 10), the parents of a 19-year-old girl with cancer ask a nurse not to tell the girl that she has cancer and is dying. The nurse agrees. But what if the girl had asked the nurse about her prognosis? What if the girl had told the nurse that she had a poor relationship with her parents because they found it hard to recognise her need for independence?

Considering stories in this way can help participants develop awareness of their own attitudes and beliefs and a sense of their professional and personal selves. It is helpful for participants to register how they feel about different options and to try to explain why they feel as they do.

Considering consequences

Reflection provides an opportunity to look at and compare the possible consequences of different actions. This too may involve 'what if', but the aim here is to consider possible outcomes rather than to explore feelings and attitudes.

For example, in Story 4 (page 10), a nurse agreed not to tell a patient that her cancer was terminal. What might the consequences have been if she had not agreed to withhold the information and had spoken to the patient? What might the consequences have been for the patient, and for her parents?

In Story 1 (page 7), a patient in intensive care says that she no longer wants any nursing care. What might be the consequences of meeting her request?

In Story 10 (page 26), a health visitor decides not to share her concerns with a mother about her baby's development. What might the consequences be for the woman? What might the consequences be if the health visitor shares her concerns?

Sometimes it is helpful to consider the best or worst possible consequences. In Story 14 (page 37), for example, nurses feel it is best to discharge a man to a nursing home, despite his family's wish to care for him at home. What might the worst possible outcome have been if, against their better judgement, they had sent him home to his family?

Making compromises

There is no answer to most of the difficulties described in Chapter 1 but practical moral compromises are usually possible. It is important that participants have an opportunity to consider and voice their feelings about such compromises.

This process may lead participants to identify issues that they wish to discuss with their managers. It is important that managerial and organisational issues are not dismissed.

Exercises

The following exercises can be used with small groups of between eight and sixteen people. They can help give a session structure, provide relief from simply 'sitting and talking', and provide stimulation. Some of the exercises are designed to develop awareness of the self and of others; others are designed to develop relevant skills such as listening skills.

All these exercises need careful facilitation. All should be explained to the group beforehand and carefully processed afterwards.

The nurse–patient/client relationship

Time estimate: 20–30 minutes

Aim: To encourage participants to become aware of the nature of their relationships with patients or clients, and especially of the extent to which they really 'know' a client.

What's needed: Paper and pencils; flipchart paper and pens.

Set up: Work individually, in pairs and in the larger group.

Leading the exercise:

Ask each participant to think of a patient or client for whom they are currently caring or whom they have cared for recently. Working individually, participants should write down what they know about that patient/client. Their list should include both facts about the patient's history, condition and personal circumstances, and also an assessment of the patient's character and needs. Everything that is known about the client should be included, however trivial. This work should

The majority of the exercises described here are taken or adapted from: Kohner N and Leftwich A. *Pregnancy Loss and the Death of a Baby. A Training Pack for Professionals.* Cambridge: National Extension College, 1995.

be done quickly, in note form. It is important not to mention names. Allow about five minutes for this part of the exercise.

Now ask each participant to find a partner – preferably one who does not know the patient or client in question. Each participant describes their client to their partner, using the written list as a prompt. The aim is to separate out known facts (e.g. he is 52 and married) from opinions, assumptions and guesswork (e.g. he is unhappily married). It may be helpful to use 'I know . . .' and 'I think . . .' Each person will need about five minutes to do this. Partners then swap roles to give the other person the chance to talk. *Remind participants not to use real names.*

The task of the listening partner is to question and challenge in order to clarify what is actually known about a patient or client and what is a matter of opinion. Where it is a matter of opinion, it is helpful for participants to explore and discuss within their pairs the basis of the opinion (e.g. 'I think he is unhappily married because his wife hardly ever comes in and he never speaks well of her' or 'I just get the feeling that's the way he is' or 'It's what his daughter told me.')

Finally ask everyone to return to the larger group for discussion.

Discussion points:

- How much did you find you really knew about your patient or client?
- How reliable is the evidence on which you base your opinions about your patient or client?
- How well do you consider you know your patients or clients?

Notes:

It is important that no names are mentioned in this exercise. Participants need to be reminded of the need for confidentiality: no information shared in the group should be repeated outside. The paper carrying information about clients should be destroyed at the end of the exercise.

It may sometimes to be useful to do a comparable exercise looking at a non-professional relationship (e.g. a friend). Information should still be destroyed at the end of the exercise.

Developing a philosophy of care

Time estimate: 20–30 minutes

Aim: To articulate the values that should inform care given by individual nurses and by the team, and to encourage professional commitment to those values. This exercise is also useful for team building.

What's needed: Flipchart paper, pens.

Set up: Small groups of four to six people.

Leading the exercise:

Begin by working in the large group. Invite everyone in the group to brainstorm single words or phrases describing quality care (e.g. honesty, empathy, confidential, consent, caring). Write the words up on the flipchart.

Now ask the group to divide into smaller groups of four to six people. Make sure everyone can see the words from the brainstorm. Ask each group to choose the five words from the list that they feel are most important. There are likely to be different opinions within each group, so there will have to be discussion and negotiation. Allow about ten minutes for this.

Now ask each group to draft a statement of maybe two or three short paragraphs, beginning with the words: 'We believe that the care we provide . . .'

Each group should work to produce a statement that everyone in the group can subscribe to.

Allow ten to fifteen minutes for this then return to the large group. Ask each group in turn to read out their philosophy of care and to talk about the process of writing it.

Discussion points:

- How easy or difficult was it to get agreement in the group?
- What does it mean to you to say that you 'believe' in this kind of care?
- How could a stated and agreed philosophy of care help you in your practice?

This exercise can be extended over a longer period of time and a number of separate sessions as a democratic way of developing or revising a unit or team philosophy. It is then helpful to ask someone in the group who can write clearly and well to take on the role of scribe. The involvement of users should be an important part of the process in order to check whether professional beliefs and priorities are shared and endorsed.

Why have you chosen to be a care worker?

Time estimate: 15 minutes.

Aim: To increase participants' awareness of what their choice of career tells them about themselves.

What's needed: Flipchart paper and pens.

Set up: Work in pairs.

Leading the exercise:

Explain that the purpose of the exercise is to help participants learn something about themselves as individuals, and in particular something about the relationship between their professional and personal selves.

Ask participants to work in pairs for five minutes and to discuss with a partner the following questions:

- What made you choose a career in the helping professions?

- What do you find most satisfying about the work you do?

Write these questions up on the flipchart where everyone can refer to them. Remind participants that each partner must have time to talk and listen.

Ask everyone to come back into the large group and pool their answers. Chart up the reasons that participants give, then ask for their views.

Discussion points:

● Have you learnt anything about yourself?
● Have you learnt anything about your profession?

Notes:

This exercise can help participants become more aware of what might influence their approach to practice.

Attitudes

Time estimate: 30–45 minutes.

Aim: To help participants identify ways in which their own beliefs, attitudes and feelings might sometimes influence the way they respond to ethical difficulties in their practice.

What's needed: Worksheet (see page 73) – one for each participant. Pens or pencils.

Set up: Individual work and small groups.

Leading the exercise:

Explain the purpose of the exercise. Hand out the worksheets.

Ask participants to look at the situations described on the worksheet and to think about which they would feel most uncomfortable about and find most difficult. They will need to imagine themselves in different roles/settings to be able to do this.

Ask each participant to rate the situations on a scale of 1 to 10 (1 = easiest, 10 = most difficult). Give everyone a few minutes for this.

Now put participants into groups according to which situation they found most difficult. (Everyone who has rated situation A as most difficult gathers into one group, and so on.) Allow about five minutes for participants to talk within their groups about why they found their chosen situation most difficult.

Now ask each group in turn to explain to the large group why they felt the situation they had chosen was particularly difficult. Encourage people in other groups to explain why they did *not* choose the same situation, and prompt general discussion.

Discussion points:

- What was it that you felt was especially difficult about the situation?
- What was easier (or less difficult) about the other situations?
- Having heard from the other groups, does anyone want to change their mind?
- Have you discovered anything about yourself?
- What might this mean for your practice?

Notes:

It is important to stress throughout this exercise that there are no right and wrong attitudes involved. The purpose of the exercise is for participants to learn about themselves and about how their own attitudes and feelings may affect the care they give. So for each participant the important task is to think about *why* they reacted to the situations in the way they did, and to be as honest as possible with themselves.

Participants can also learn a lot from each other so it is important to facilitate discussion well. It should become clear that people have very different views and moral stances, and this can mean that they care in different ways.

WORKSHEET

Look at the statements listed below. Decide which situation you would feel most uncomfortable with. Try to go with your gut reaction: there are no right and wrong answers. Score each situation 1 to 10 (10 = extremely uncomfortable).

1 You are caring for a woman who has breast cancer. She has been offered the choice between a lumpectomy and a mastectomy. She has been given information about these options by the consultant and has had a number of opportunities to talk. But she is finding it very hard to make the decision and is distressed. She turns to you and says, 'I don't know what to do. You decide for me.'

2 An elderly man on your ward has made a good recovery after a stroke. You are his primary nurse. He is now very keen to go home but you know that he lives alone and is unlikely to be able to care for himself. He is forgetful, often confused and unsteady on his feet. You and the rest of the team feel he should go into residential care but he is adamant that he wants to go home.

3 A ten-year-old boy has died after a week in intensive care. You have been caring for him and have got to know his family. His parents now want to take his body home until the funeral. They would like to dress him and take him in their own car. They ask you to help them do this.

4 You are a health visitor. One of your clients is a mother with two small children. When the second baby was born, she suffered severe depression and was admitted to hospital for a short time. She recovered well but now, two years later, is very depressed again. She confides in you that the doctor has prescribed anti-depressants but she doesn't want to take them. She asks you not to tell the doctor.

5 A man in his seventies who has cancer has been offered chemotherapy. He stands a good chance of recovery. He tells you that he does not want this or any treatment but wishes to be discharged. There is no doubt that he understands the implications of his decision.

A day off

Time estimate: 30 minutes.

Aim: to help participants develop awareness of themselves and of the invisible differences between people. The exercise also helps people learn what it feels like to self-disclose.

What's needed: paper and coloured pens for each participant (see below).

Set up: Individual work and in the large group.

Leading the exercise:

Explain the purpose of the exercise.

Tell the group that they have each been given an extra paid day off work. Ask each participant to think about what they would like to do with the day. They can do anything they please. Alternatively, ask participants to draw their day on a large piece of paper with coloured pens. Allow about five minutes, or longer for drawing.

Now ask each participant to describe their day, saying something about why they have chosen it. Alternatively, if the group have produced drawings, put them all up on the wall and ask each participant in turn to talk about their drawing.

End the exercise by discussing what is likely to be a wide variety of choices.

Discussion points:

- Was it easy or difficult for you to decide what to do with your day?
- Was it difficult to talk about it to the group?

Experiencing powerlessness

Time estimate: 5 minutes.

Aim: To identify what it feels like when someone else is in control.

This is a simple, funny exercise which can be used as an ice-breaker or to liven up a group. It can also establish a good base for work on empowerment.

Set up: Work in pairs and in the large group.

Leading the exercise:

Ask participants to find a partner: one person is A and the other B. A leads B round the room while B keeps his or her eyes tightly closed. A must take care of B and make sure he or she doesn't collide with anything or anyone. After a few minutes, A and B change over.

Ask everyone to sit down again in a circle to talk about the exercise. It may be helpful to chart up the feelings that are expressed.

Discussion points:

- What did it feel like to hand over control to someone else?
- What helped?
- What did it feel like to be the one with the responsibility?

Notes:

Although some participants are likely to have done this exercise before, it is worth repeating it. It can help participants bring some immediate feelings to consideration of power and control.

After further work, participants can be asked to repeat this exercise. This time, the person with their eyes closed can choose what they would like to do (walk to the other end of the room, sit or lie down, walk out of the door, put on their coat . . .). The person leading must help them to do it. Return to the large group to discuss whether the feelings were different this time.

Remember a time when you felt powerless

Time estimate: 15 minutes.

Aim: To increase participants' awareness of what it is like to be powerless/have no control.

Set up: Work in pairs.

Leading the exercise:

Ask participants to find a partner: one person is A, the other B. Ask both to try to remember a time when they felt powerless or not in control. If this is difficult, prompt participants with some possible situations – such as their first day at school, or their first day in a new job.

A talks to B about this time, focusing particularly on *what it felt like* to be powerless. After about five minutes, they change over and B talks while A listens. Warn everyone when time is nearly up.

Ask everyone to come back into the large group for discussion.

Many people are surprised by the extent to which their normal ability to ask questions and control situations can be affected by new, strange or difficult situations.

Professional roles – How are we seen? How would we like to be seen?

Time estimate: 15 minutes.

Aim: To help participants consider what is expected of them and what they expect of themselves in their professional roles.

What's needed: Two pieces of flipchart paper and a pen for each group.

Set up: Small groups of four to six people.

Leading the exercise:

Ask participants to split into small groups of four to six people. Each group needs two pieces of flipchart paper and a pen. Ask each group to list on one sheet of paper how they feel they are seen by members of the public. Then, on a separate sheet, ask them to list how they would like to be seen. They will need about ten minutes. Warn everyone when time is nearly up.

Ask everyone to come back into the large group and put the lists up on the wall. Ask a spokesperson from each group to run through the lists and explain their discussion. Ask everyone for their thoughts and comments.

Discussion points:

- What is the relationship between how participants *would like* to be seen and how they feel they *are* seen?
- To what extent do they themselves feel they should be able to cope with ethical difficulties and dilemmas in their practice?
- To what extent do they feel patients or clients feel they should be able to cope?
- What does this mean for their practice, especially when they find they don't know what to do?
- What would it mean for how they are seen if they were known to have behaved unethically (e.g. lying, withholding information, treating without consent, etc.)?

Notes:

The expectations that others have of professionals and their own expectations of themselves can make a formidable (and sometimes unrealistic) list. It can help to recognise that we all have limits.

Chapter 4

Summary of stories

1 *Against her wishes (page 7)*

A patient who has been in special care for some time states clearly that she no longer wants any nursing care.

Discussion points

- What reasons might there be (if any) for not agreeing to a patient's requests or wishes?
- How do you think you might feel as a patient if you asked for something and were denied it?
- Do patients have the right to dictate the care they are given? If not, why not?
- Do patients have the right to refuse care and/or treatment?
- How would you feel if a patient refused care that you felt was in their best interests?

2 *'Get me home' (page 8)*

An elderly woman who has had severe heart failure wants to be discharged home. To keep well, she will need to take her tablets and limit her fluid intake. It seems unlikely that she will do either. Should she be discharged?

Discussion points

- Does the patient have a right to be discharged, even if this involves risk?
- What is the extent of a nurse's responsibility to protect a patient from harm?
- What could you do in this situation in order to meet the woman's need to go home and yet minimise risk?

3 'Tell me what to do' (page 9)

Anne has four small children and her partner has left her. She is pregnant. At first she decides she will have a termination, then wavers. She cannot decide what to do and is in distress. She asks her health visitor to make her decision for her.

Discussion points

- Should the health visitor give advice or should she hold back, saying it has to be Anne's decision? Give your reasons.
- The health visitor knows Anne's personal situation and has an established and good relationship with her. Are there factors that might justify her expressing an opinion about what Anne should do? Would your thinking about the situation change if the health visitor did not know Anne well?
- What might be the short and long-term consequences of the health visitor giving, or not giving, advice?
- In what circumstances, if any, should a health visitor or nurse make a decision on a client's behalf?
- Do you think that Anne's partner has any rights in this situation?

4 'She never asked . . .' (page 10)

The parents of a 19-year-old girl ask that she is not told that she has terminal cancer. The nurse agrees to their request.

Discussion points

- Do you consider the nurse's agreement not to give the girl information about her illness is justifiable? On what grounds?
- Do patients have a right to know that they are dying?
- Suppose the nurse had decided to tell the girl that she was dying. What might the consequences have been? Consider both the girl's possible feelings and her parents'.
- This nurse's response might have been different if she had found the girl's parents less sympathetic. How much is practice influenced by positive or negative feelings about patients/clients and their families? Is it right that it should be influenced in this way?

5 An open door (page 12)

A story from a dementia unit with a locked door. The nurses have made a decision to open the door if patients wish to go out, and to go out with them.

Discussion points

- What are your feelings about responding to patients in this way?
- If a patient asks to leave the ward, on what grounds can you justify not allowing him or her to do so? How do you feel about this justification?
- If a patient asks to leave the ward and is prevented from doing so, what does this mean for the nurse-patient relationship? How does the nurse-patient relationship change if the door is opened and the patient is accompanied out?
- Are there any considerations to be taken into account besides the rights and needs of the patients?

6 Permissible or indefensible? (page 13)

A man admitted to an acute medical ward is both psychotic and physically ill. He marches up and down the ward and creates confusion. It is essential to calm him down and so the nurse tranquillises him without his knowledge by putting drugs in his tea.

The same nurse also tells how he feels as the relative of a patient who is being treated in the same way. Although he feels it is indefensible to treat patients in this way, as a nurse he can understand it, as a relative he feels appalled.

Discussion points

- Do you consider that tranquillising patients without their knowledge or consent can be justified? On what grounds?
- Following an incident like this, what could nurses on the ward do to avoid or mitigate similar difficulties in the future?
- This nurse's feelings as a relative were very different to his feelings as a professional. How might his feelings as a relative influence his professional practice in the future?

7 Duty or interference? (page 14)

A man comes in to an accident and emergency department. He is drunk. After treatment he leaves, intending to drive home. Without telling the man, the nurse informs the police.

Discussion points

- Do you consider it was right or wrong of the nurse to pass on this information? Give your reasons.
- Consider and decide how you would act in this situation. Give your reasons.

8 Questions of trust and judgement (page 23)

A nurse on night duty cares for a woman who has been beaten by her husband. He has to spend a lot of time with her in order to gain her trust. She is grateful for his care and help and when they are alone, she embraces him.

Discussion points

- The nurse worked hard to create a relationship with this patient in order to be able to help her. Nevertheless, did he exceed his responsibilities? How much is emotional care a legitimate and necessary part of a nurse's job?
- How do you decide whether to believe/trust a patient? How do you encourage a patient to trust you?
- How could the nurse have protected himself but still helped his patient?

9 What did she want? (page 25)

A pregnant woman tells her midwife that when she is in labour, she does not want to have an epidural. She writes this down. But when she is in labour, she demands an epidural. The midwife makes a decision not to meet this request but to try to help the woman through her labour without an epidural.

Discussion points

- What role did clinical experience and professional judgement play in the midwife's decision to not to give the epidural? What other factors may have influenced her decision?
- What might your feelings have been as the client in this story?
- In the relationship between a nurse or midwife and a client, are there responsibilities on both sides? What, if any, do you consider are the responsibilities of the client?
- How well can a nurse/midwife know a client or patient?
- Do you feel that the client's gratitude justifies the midwife's decision?

10 'I didn't want to worry her' (page 26)

A health visitor has a client, a new mother who worries a lot. The mother has noticed that her baby is slow to sit up and asks the health visitor whether there is a problem. The health visitor is herself concerned but feels it is too early to say anything. In response to the mother's question, the health visitor says that she does not think there is any need to worry.

Discussion points

- Do you feel the health visitor's response was justifiable? On what grounds?
- What does the health visitor's decision not to share her concern mean for her relationship with this client?
- How do you think the health visitor's decision not to express her own anxieties might affect her relationship with this mother in the future?

11 A sense of betrayal (page 27)

A health visitor has an established relationship with a mother, Jean, who has a violent partner. On a home visit, the health visitor notices that Jean's young daughter is bruised. She talks about this to Jean who confirms that her partner has hit the little girl. Jean asks the health visitor not to report the bruising to the social services. Anxious to maintain Jean's trust, the health visitor agrees. But later she changes her mind and reports what she has seen.

Discussion points

- What factors would you consider in trying to decide whether or not to report a case like this?
- The health visitor describes her feelings about her relationship with Jean. What might Jean's feelings be? How do you think these feelings might be changed by the health visitor reporting her child's bruising?
- What might the consequences have been if the health visitor had not mentioned the bruising to the mother at all and had gone straight to the social services?

12 Taking sides (page 35)

A 14-year-old girl is brought into an accident and emergency department having been kicked in the stomach at school. The girl tells the nurse she is pregnant but asks her not to tell her mother. The nurse agrees not to tell.

Discussion points

- What are the arguments to support the nurse's decision to take the girl's side?
- What are the arguments in favour of telling the mother about her daughter's pregnancy?
- What is the nurse's responsibility in this situation?

13 For whose good? (page 36)

An elderly lady with dementia wants to go home. Her son, who cares for her, is ill as a result of the stress and work of caring for her. He feels he cannot cope and needs a break; she wants and needs to be at home.

Discussion points

- What is the role of the primary nurse in this situation? How can she best support her patient?
- What responsibility, if any, does the nurse have towards the son?
- Are there occasions when the needs of a patient's family could be considered more important than the patient's needs?

14 'We thought we knew best' (page 37)

After a number of strokes, Steve needs long-term care. His family want to care for him but the nurses feel they may not be able to give him the care he needs. They make a decision to move Steve to a nursing home. Steve makes it clear that he does not want to be in the home: he walks out. His family then take him in and care for him successfully.

Discussion points

- Was it justifiable to persuade the family to accept a decision they did not want? On what grounds?
- What is your assessment of the risk of sending Steve home to live with his family? What might the consequences have been?
- Are there occasions when the needs of a patient's family could be considered more important than the patient's needs?

15 Whose advocate? (page 38)

A long-term patient in intensive care develops infections which the medical staff do not want to investigate or treat. The nurse caring for the woman decides to speak to her husband and advises him to insist that his wife has treatment if that is what he wants.

Discussion points

- As the patient's advocate, should the nurse take the side of the patient or family, even, if necessary, in opposition to medical staff?
- How can a nurse best fulfil his or her role as the patient's advocate if the patient is unable to communicate? Is it acceptable to use

a relative or friend of the patient as an indicator of the patient's values? What are the risks involved in doing this?

● In this nurse's place, how would you approach the husband and what would you wish to discuss with him?

16 Breaking bad news (page 43)

After the death of a man in accident and emergency, a nurse has to break the news to his wife. To his astonishment, she is not upset but relieved. The man's mother also comes to the hospital. The wife asks the nurse not to tell her mother-in-law that she is in the hospital, and to tell her that she is grieving, although she is not. The nurse agrees to lie on the wife's behalf.

Discussion points

● The nurse made a decision based on intuition. What were the risks involved?
● Do you feel it is acceptable to use intuition in this way?
● Do you feel it was the nurse's responsibility to help the wife in the way he did?
● Can you devise any alternative strategies for handling this situation?

17 A vulnerable client (page 45)

A woman with a mild learning disability has developed a relationship with the taxi driver who takes her to and from a bingo session each week. The taxi driver wants the relationship to develop further; the woman does not. The community nurse, who supports the woman, has to decide whether (and how) to intervene.

Discussion points

● Do you think that someone with a mild learning disability has the same right to the same degree of autonomy as someone with no disability?
● What do you consider to be the nurse's responsibility in this situation?
● How could the nurse intervene most helpfully?

18 For her good but against her will? (page 46)

A woman with severe manic depression is admitted to a psychiatric ward, rational but very depressed. She has a history of self–harm. She wants to leave and is assessed. It is decided that she should not be sectioned and should be free to leave. But the nurse caring for her is very worried about her. She decides to put her on continuous supervision so that she cannot leave, even though she has not been sectioned.

Later, the woman tells the nurse that she was glad that she had not let her leave as she had intended to kill herself.

Discussion points

● Since the woman was assessed as rational, was it justifiable for the nurse to decide to prevent her from leaving the ward? On what grounds?
● Whose responsibility was it to ensure this woman received the right treatment?

19 Problems of priorities (page 47)

A nurse's observations about the difficulty of deciding priorities in nursing care.

Discussion points

● On what basis should priorities for nursing care be decided?
● To what extent can, or should, these priorities be set by the individual practitioner?
● How can you balance the time you give to visible and invisible care?

20 The tea trolley (page 48)

The tea trolley is brought to the ward every afternoon and patients are asked if they would like a cup of tea. But patients who, for whatever reason, do not respond do not receive a cup of tea.

Discussion points

- Identify exactly what is unethical about this situation.
- Whose responsibility is it to rectify this situation?
- What kind of changes are needed? How can they be brought about?

21 If only . . . (page 48)

A midwife cares for a pregnant woman with a history of depression. The woman fears that she will become acutely depressed after her baby is born, as her sister did. Her sister was treated with ECT and the woman is terrified that this will also happen to her.

She becomes psychotic postnatally and is admitted to a psychiatric unit. She begs the midwife to ensure she is not given ECT. The midwife supports her and says that as far as she is able she will ensure this. She is treated with drugs. Three months later, she commits suicide.

Discussion points

- The midwife who told this story felt that the woman did not want to die. Would your thoughts about the story be different if the woman had said that she *did* want to die?
- Is it justifiable to ignore a client's requests if you believe that complying would be harmful to them or to others?
- What was the midwife's responsibility towards her client in this situation?

References

1. Department of Health. *Caring for People.* London: HMSO, 1989

2. Department of Health. *The Patient's Charter.* London: HMSO, 1991

3. NHS Management Executive. *A Vision for the Future. The nursing, midwifery and health visiting contribution to health and health care.* London: Department of Health, 1993

4. Department of Health. *Changing Childbirth.* London: HMSO, 1993

5. Seedhouse D. *Ethics. The heart of health care.* Chichester: John Wiley & Sons, 1988

6. Gillon R. Medical ethics: four principles plus attention to scope. *British Medical Journal* 1994; 309:184–8

7. UKCC. *Code of Conduct for the Nurse, Midwife and Health Visitor.* London: United Kingdom Central Council for Nursing, Midwifery and Health Visiting, 1992

8. UKCC. *The Scope of Professional Practice.* London: United Kingdom Central Council for Nursing, Midwifery and Health Visiting, 1992

9. Hunt G (ed). *Ethical Issues in Nursing.* London: Routledge, 1994

Further reading

Ashworth P D, Longmate M A, Morrison P. Patient participation: its meaning and significance in the context of caring. *Journal of Advanced Nursing* 1992; 17:1430–9

Beisecker A E, Beisecker T D. Using metaphors to characterise doctor-patient relationships: paternalism versus consumerism. *Health Communication* 1993; 5(1):41–58

Benner P, Wrubel J. *The Primacy of Caring.* Menlo Park (CA): Addison-Wesley, 1989

Biley F. Some determinants that effect patient participation in decision-making about nursing care. *Journal of Advanced Nursing* 1992; 17:414–21

Campbell A V. *Moderated Love: A theology of professional care.* London: SPCK, 1984

Copperman J, Morrison P. *We Thought We Knew . . . Involving patients in nursing practice.* London: King's Fund Centre, 1995

Curtin L, Flaherty M J. *Nursing Ethics. Theories and pragmatics.* Bowie (Maryland): Robert J Brady Co, 1982

Downie R S, Calman K C. *Healthy Respect. Ethics in health care.* 2nd edition. Oxford: Oxford University Press, 1994

Gillon R. Medical ethics: four principles plus attention to scope. *British Medical Journal* 1994; 309:184–8

Gillon R, Lloyd A (eds). *Principles of Health Care Ethics.* Chichester: John Wiley & Sons, 1994

Glenister D. Patient participation in psychiatric services: a literature review and proposal for a research strategy. *Journal of Advanced Nursing* 1992; 19:802–11

Hogg C. *Beyond the Patient's Charter.* London: Health Rights, 1993

Holm S. 'What is wrong with compliance? *Journal of Medical Ethics* 1993; 19(2):108–10

Hunt G (ed). *Ethical Issues in Nursing.* London: Routledge, 1994

Hunt G. What is nursing ethics? *Nurse Education Today* 1994; 12:323–8

Illich I. *Limits to Medicine.* Harmondsworth: Penguin, 1978

Jackson J. Telling the truth. *Journal of Medical Ethics* 1991; 17(1):5–9, and Bakhurst D. On lying and deceiving. *Journal of Medical Ethics* 1992; 18(2):63–6

McIver S. *Obtaining the Views of Users of Health Services.* London: King's Fund Centre, 1991

Robinson K, Vaughan B. *Knowledge for Nursing Practice.* Oxford: Butterworth Heinemann, 1992

Saunders P. Encouraging patients to take part in their own care. *Nursing Times* 1995; 91(9): 42–3

Seedhouse D. *Ethics. The heart of health care.* Chichester: John Wiley & Sons, 1988

Seedhouse D, Cribb A (eds). *Changing Health Care.* Chichester: John Wiley & Sons, 1988

Shackley P, Ryan M. What is the role of the consumer in health care? *Journal of Social Policy* 1994; 23(4):517–41

Stewart M *et al. Patient-Centered Medicine. Transforming the clinical method.* Thousand Oaks (CA): Sage Publications, 1995

Tschudin V. *Ethics in Nursing: The caring relationship.* 2nd edition, London: Butterworth Heinemann, 1992

Tschudin V. *Ethics: Nurses and patients.* Harrow: Scutari Press, 1993

UKCC. *Guidelines for Professional Practice.* London: United Kingdom Central Council for Nursing, Midwifery and Health Visiting, 1996

Wear A N, Brahams D. To treat or not to treat: the legal, ethical and therapeutic implications of treatment refusal. *Journal of Medical Ethics* 1991; 17(3):131–5

Wreen M J. Autonomy, religious values, and refusal of lifesaving medical treatment. *Journal of Medical Ethics* 1991; 17(3):124–30

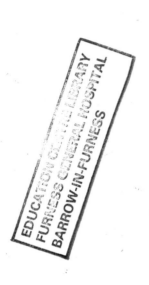